Segregation, Poverty, and Mortality in Urban African Americans

Segregation, Poverty, and Mortality in Urban African Americans

Anthony P. Polednak, Ph.D.

State of Connecticut
Department of Public Health

New York   Oxford
OXFORD UNIVERSITY PRESS
1997

Oxford University Press

Oxford   New York
Athens   Auckland   Bangkok   Bogota
Bombay   Buenos Aires   Calcutta   Cape Town
Dar es Salaam   Delhi   Florence   Hong Kong   Istanbul
Karachi   Kuala Lumper   Madras   Madrid
Melbourne   Mexico City   Nairobi   Paris
Singapore   Taipei   Tokyo   Toronto

and associated companies in
Berlin   Ibadan

Library of Congress Cataloging-in-Publication Data
Polednak, Anthony P.
Segregation, poverty, and mortality in urban African Americans /
Anthony P. Polednak.
p.   cm.   Includes bibliographical references and index.
ISBN 0-19-511165-6
1. Afro-Americans—Segregation.
2. Afro-Americans—Mortality.
3. Afro-Americans—Health and hygiene.
4. Afro-Americans—Social conditions—1975–
I. Title.
E185.86.P64   1997   305.896'073—dc20   96-27947

9 8 7 6 5 4 3 2 1

Printed in the United States of America
on acid-free paper

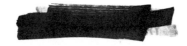

Preface

My interest in the potential impact of segregation on the health of blacks (African Americans) was stimulated by the chance reading of an article in a sociological journal (Massey and Denton, 1987) dealing with time trends in black–white residential segregation. The higher degree of segregation of U.S. whites from blacks than from other racial and ethnic groups, and the obvious association between segregation and overall quality of life, suggested that segregation might be related in complex ways to the health of blacks. My first work in this area, dealing with infant mortality (Polednak, 1991), was done without awareness of previous efforts to examine the association between segregation and black infant mortality rates (Yankauer, 1950; LaVeist, 1989).

This book brings together data from several studies that have examined the association between degree of black–white residential segregation and mortality rates for blacks in selected U.S. urban areas, with some control (statistically) for variation in black–white disparities in social class. It also presents previously unpublished analyses that include additional calendar years of mortality data, along with data from the 1990 U.S. census. These analyses are useful mainly in generating hypotheses to be explored by analytic studies that include information on individuals. The goal of these analyses is to increase interest, on the part of sociologists and epidemiologists, in what might be called the "epidemiology of American apartheid." This extends the work of sociologists Massey and Denton on *American Apartheid* (1993) into the area of public health. Mortality rates are used not only because of the availability of data but also because they demonstrate the underprivileged status of blacks. By tradition in public health, infant mortality rates have been used as an index of social progress.

The goal is to call greater attention to the high mortality rates for blacks in many urban areas, as a reflection of their unique experience with discrimination. Such attempts recognize bell hooks's perceptive comments (1995) about the hopelessness (for blacks) of adopting the role of victim, despite obvious victimization, and understandable black ambivalence with regard to integration and "assimilation." Despite these dilemmas, the epidemiology of American apartheid should prove not only challenging but rewarding, in terms of its implications for social and health policy.

The intended audience includes sociologists, especially medical sociologists, who are likely to be familiar with the issue of segregation but not with its relevance to the health of African Americans. Epidemiologists are another potential audience because they have recently turned to the study of racism and health, although epidemiologic studies have not dealt specifically with black–white segregation and health. This book could stimulate some epidemiologists to include variables related to segregation in their studies.

Sociologists and epidemiologists, along with psychologists, will be familiar with the uses and limits of the statistical method (multiple linear regression) used in the analyses of poverty rates and level of segregation as predictors of variation in black mortality rates among large U.S. metropolitan areas (Chapter 5). However, in an effort to maximize readability for a wider audience, tables with regression models have been placed in the Appendix, along with detailed tabulations of data for large numbers of metropolitan areas.

Psychologists interested in racism or related areas could be important collaborators with sociologists and epidemiologists in studies of the epidemiology of American apartheid. Readers working in social policy and health policy areas, including urban issues, should find some relevant materials, especially in the final chapter.

For general readers, this work fits within the framework of Swedish economist G. Myrdal's "American dilemma" thesis (1944) that the "American creed" of equality of opportunity and freedom from discrimination remains unfulfilled. Little background in statistics is needed to read most of this book, and explanations of correlation coefficients and linear regression (if needed) can be found in texts on basic statistics.

Contents

Segregation, Poverty, and Mortality in Urban African Americans

1

Introduction:
Purpose and Plan

Sociology and Epidemiology: An Interface

Sociology and American Institutions

Sociology is concerned with the development of various social institutions. The British historian and economist R.H. Tawney noted that "every generation regards as natural the institutions to which it is accustomed." In the history of blacks in America, the relevant institutions are slavery (the South's self-proclaimed "peculiar institution"), postemancipation legalized segregation, and post-civil-rights-era de facto segregation. The archaeologist V.G. Childe (1892–1957), who traced the prehistoric record of human social-technological "revolutions" (including the "urban revolution"), observed that social traditions are shaped by individuals and communities, and the "institutions of oppression" are "not fixed and immutable" (Childe, 1951).

D.L. Lewis began his Pulitzer Prize–winning biography of black sociologist W.E.B. Du Bois (1868–1963) with an account of the August 1963 civil rights march on Washington, during which the announcement of the death of Du Bois (the "old man") was made to the audience of more than 250,000. Du Bois died in Ghana, not while on a visit but as a citizen and resident for several years after abandoning hope for social and economic equality for blacks in America. During Du Bois' life, many changes had occurred in American institutions that affected blacks. Born 5 years after the Emancipation Proclamation was issued, he absorbed much of the experience of slavery from the memories of its survivors. The first African American to receive a Harvard doctorate, a founder of the NAACP, and "the premier architect of the civil rights movement in the United States" (Lewis, 1993), Du Bois wrote extensively on the slave trade, slave culture, and the persisting detrimental influences of slavery on blacks. Du Bois lived until the advent, albeit not the culmination, of the civil rights era of the 1960s.

3

Du Bois' emigration to Africa is ironic when considered in the historical context of the "colonization" movement of the nineteenth century. Many abolitionist whites (including Presidents Lincoln and Grant) and Congress planned to transport blacks, voluntarily (according to Lincoln) or otherwise, to various countries including Africa. Some black intellectuals, down to Du Bois and S. Carmichael, supported various forms of colonization. Earlier, even F. Douglass, although a staunch advocate of an integrated, "color blind" society, had "toyed" with it (Freehling, 1994). Instead of the "colonization" of blacks, an internal "colony" model of blacks has emerged (Henry, 1990), along with calls for blacks to "decolonize" themselves from a "color caste" society that devalues blackness (especially higher degrees of black skin color) (hooks, 1995).

The complex changes in Du Bois' attitudes and writings over his long life are symbolic of the continuing dilemmas and ambivalences some American blacks have with regard to forms of integration or (to use the more extreme term) "assimilation" that deny the value of black cultural heritage and devalue blackness itself into a society plagued by both white racism and the denial of its existence. The life of Malcolm X, strikingly different from that of Du Bois, demonstrated a different evolution. At the end of his short life, Malcolm X envisioned the potential benefits of combatting white racism and working with whites. The place of Malcolm X, the "great prophet of black rage" (West, 1994), is recognized among those black thinkers who inform blacks about "decolonization" and resistance (hooks, 1995). However, the views of Malcolm X and of other black nationalists betray a fear of "cultural hybridity" or an African-American culture that has always been a unique mixture of elements from African, European, and Amerindian sources (West, 1994). West (1994) argued that black self-esteem, self-love, and self-determination can be accepted without embracing black nationalist ideology.

hooks (1995) has associated black nationalism with an unrealistic, utopian vision of Africa before the advent of white colonialism, and separatism was rejected in favor of the hope of forging a new version of M.L. King Jr.'s "beloved community" that does not require that African Americans surrender ties to their African cultural heritage. Black "self-determination" (hooks, 1995) recalls Du Bois' ideas on strengthening the black community economically, socially, and morally, with the incorporation of pre-colonial African cultural and social values. These ideas were unacceptable to the NAACP, which he left in 1934 (although he later returned, before the final breach) (Stuckey, 1987). However, these ideas, including the nurturing of black schools and colleges as well as black communities, are enjoying a revival among black scholars, as well as increased interest among anthropologists (Harrison, 1995).

While accepting integration as a long-range goal for blacks, Du Bois (in *The Conservation of Races*, 1897) described a "racial two-ness" reminiscent of F. Douglass' "nation within a nation." *Two Nations* (Hacker, 1992, 1995) was subtitled *Black and White, Separate, Hostile, Unequal*, paraphrasing the "separate and unequal" black and white "societies" idea in the Kerner Commission report on civil disturbances during the 1960s (Kerner, 1968). Hacker's tone was decidedly pessimistic, and the preface warned the reader not to "look for a closing chapter with proposals for reducing discrimination and ending preju-dice," because "racial tensions serve too many important purposes to be easily ameliorated" (Hacker, 1995). While recognizing the authenticity of Hacker's depiction, hooks (1995), in *Killing Rage: Ending Racism,* warned against a sense of hopelessness in race relations and argued for self-determination by black communities without abandoning the attempt to reach out to other groups.

The "purposes" or "functions" of the institution of *de facto* segregation have been described by Massey and Denton (1993). These sociologists depicted segregation as an "institution" deliberately maintained by the majority for the chief purpose of attempting to isolate blacks and the social and economic prob-lems perceived as being associated with ghettos. They also argued that the importance of segregation as a factor in reinforcing the low social and economic status of blacks, as well as in fostering the "social pathology" of inner cities, is not adequately acknowledged. Indeed, the word *segregation* itself is often miss-ing from social and political discussions, except for school desegregation issues at the local level. The myth that white racism, as depicted by Hacker and by black scholars, does not exist (hooks, 1995) is itself symptomatic of the denial involved in the "disease" of racism.

Both social class and residential segregation result in social stratification, which is a sociological issue. The persistence of both black–white segregation and higher poverty rates among blacks in the United States results in the tendency for urban blacks of all social classes to be concentrated in high-poverty areas or areas of extreme poverty (called *poverty areas* by some sociologists) (Chapter 3). These urban black populations, while comprising only a small fraction of all "poor" persons, strongly influence the debate about the causes of and cures for poverty, the "urban underclass," and the "welfare system."

The black hospital movement, which flourished from around 1920 to 1945, arose not only as a reaction to segregated medical care of grossly inferior quality for blacks in existing hospitals but also from "the African-American commu-nity's longstanding tradition of providing for its members" (Gamble, 1995). This is part of the "dialectic" between opposing segregation and nurturing the black community. It may be viewed historically as part of a larger conflict between "multicultural diversification" and "national homogenization" in which some fractions of immigrants of each ethnic group gave up the fight for integration and (often reinforced by the wishes of the majority) returned to their homelands (Freehling, 1994). However, the institutions of slavery and extreme segregation made the black experience in the United States different from that of the immigrant groups.

In *An American Dilemma,* Swedish economist G. Myrdal (1944) proposed that the situation for blacks represented an incongruity between American values, or an "American creed" of equality of opportunity, and the realities of discrimination and segregation. Sociology is also concerned with incongruities between value systems and social realities. Alexis de Tocqueville's classic nineteenth-century work, *Democracy in America,* is often cited by sociologists with regard not only to its description of the American values of individualism and individual responsibility that continue to affect attitudes regarding the causes of poverty and low social class but also to its prediction that the problem of integration of blacks into the larger society would persist (Gans, 1990; Hacker, 1995).

While not limited to blacks or minorities, the sociological concept of an "American dream package" (Perrucci and Knudsen, 1983) of equal opportunity for success, embedded deeply in the American ethos and value system, influences debates about poverty, welfare, and equal opportunity for racial and ethnic groups. Popular ("pop") sociology (Gans, 1990) has had an impact on societal attitudes and political decision making, especially with regard to the theory of the detrimental effects of "welfare" on individuals (Murray, 1984). Less media attention has been given to sociological and ethnographic studies that have documented the lives of the uninsured "working poor" whose savings are suddenly lost due to the costs of catastrophic illness or of elderly persons surviving only on social security benefits but in need of food stamps and nursing home care not covered by Medicare (Rank, 1994).

Also receiving minimal recognition in popular and political debates is the discrimination against blacks in hiring and other areas as "structural" impediments to achieving economic self-sufficiency. Sociologist J. Quadagno (1994) has argued that white racism, in its attempt to maintain discrimination in housing and jobs, has influenced the entire history of welfare programs and the failure to address the problems of inner cities in America. Work by sociologists has shown the importance of racial discrimination in limiting job opportunities for blacks living in inner cities and such economic issues as the lack of strong black labor markets in understanding black–white disparities in poverty rates (Stafford and Ladner 1990).

Socioeconomic Epidemiology and Beyond

The underprivileged status of the American black population is demonstrated by lower social status relative to that of whites. Another aspect of this status, which involves public health and its basic science (epidemiology), is the persistence of higher death rates for blacks than whites in the United States, especially in certain urban areas. The use of mortality rates as an indicator of underprivileged status for blacks was advanced by Kitagawa and Hauser's classic work *Differential Mortality in the United States* (1973). Their concept of "socioeconomic epidemiology" combined the sociological concept of social class with epidemiologic interests in the distribution of disease and death rates by showing the "underprivileged" status of blacks with regard to mortality rates. More recently, epidemiologists have begun to consider the measurement and applications of social class concepts (Liberatos et al., 1988), a realm previously reserved for sociologists.

While Kitagawa and Hauser (1973) described differences in mortality rates between blacks and whites and variations in death rates by social class and region within the United States, they did not consider the potential role of segregation and other forms of discrimination. The possible relationships between black–white residential segregation and the health of black populations have received limited attention by epidemiologists, who study the distribution of disease according to characteristics of person, place, and time. Similarly, while long involved in research dealing with the description and explanation of de facto segregation in the United States, American sociologists (even medical sociologists) have rarely used epidemiologic methods to assess the health consequences of poverty and segregation for the African-American population.

A review of historical data on black–white differences in mortality in the United States concluded that such differences could not be understood by considering only social class differences as the "ultimate determinants" and that, despite difficulties in documenting the mechanisms involved, racial discrimination affected these differentials (Ewbank, 1987). While not specifically mentioned by Ewbank, discrimination in housing is the major cause of black–white segregation, which has an impact on the quality of life for blacks and may be related to the health of blacks in complex ways. The main purpose of this book is to stimulate dialogue and research in this area.

Massey and Denton (1993) chose the title *American Apartheid* because of similarities between the social institutions of South Africa and America with regard to blacks. This suggests that segregation may be inimical to the health of African Americans, as shown for South Africans. This book addresses the question of the degree to which black–white residential segregation is associated with the health status of urban African Americans and considers possible explanations for any associations found. This issue is raised cautiously, in view of the dilemmas mentioned in this chapter, and the dilemma of the hopelessness of individual blacks' adopting the role of "victim" while calling attention to their obvious victimization (hooks, 1995). Stressing the problems of inner-city black neighborhoods without close attention to the causes underlying these problems may contribute to the attempt to "ghettoize" the social problems (such as excessive materialism and individualism, crime, drugs, and violence) that also plague the larger, "mainstream" society.

Nevertheless, the tradition of public health includes the identification of persons, groups, or geographic areas at relatively high risk for adverse health outcomes. Complex interactions would be expected among the variables of race, social class, social status, residential segregation, and health. A sociological perspective is crucial to understanding the potential impact of segregation on the health, as well as on the social class and social status, of blacks.

Conceptual Framework and Plan of the Book

The conceptual framework for this book is outlined in Figure 1-1; further details are developed later. Briefly, white prejudice results in discrimination. The well-recognized progression is from prejudice (attitudes) to discrimination (behavior), including discrimination in housing. *Prejudice* or "pre-judgement" of individuals based on their membership in a group is an "avertive or hostile attitude" based on perceived "objectionable qualities" ascribed to a group "without sufficient warrant" (Allport, 1969). *Racism* is a composite term that

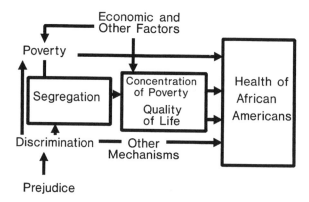

Figure 1-1. Conceptual framework.

includes "prejudice, negative attitudes and beliefs about other groups," and "discrimination" or "differential treatment" based solely on race or ethnicity (Williams et al., 1994). "Unequal treatment of equals" on the basis of perceived racial affiliation is a good, short definition of discrimination (Fix and Struyk, 1993). Racism is institutionalized or widespread discrimination on the basis of race or ethnicity. Any form of race recognition based on biological or genetic differences is sometimes regarded as racism, but, in the absence of ranking of groups or of beliefs in inherent "racial inferiority," this would more aptly be called *race consciousness* (Jaynes and Williams, 1989, Appendix A).

Racism involves prejudice transformed into "the exercise of power against a racial group" judged to be "inferior" by individuals and institutions, whether intentional or unintentional (Jones, 1981; Ponterotto and Pedersen, 1993), or into institutionalized "racial-power inequality" (Feagin, 1991). In some schemes, racism cannot exist for a group that has little power over another (Hacker, 1995), but opinions differ on this point. C. West (1994) referred to "black supremacy" in connection with the black nationalism movement.

Discrimination, especially according to "structural" theories of poverty (Chapter 3), is a major cause of black–white disparities in income and social class. Social class, often defined by level of income and/or education, is a key variable in relation to health and mortality. However, the combination of lower social class (or higher risk of being poor) for all blacks compared with whites and persistent black–white segregation may have an impact on the quality of health for blacks. For blacks, but rarely for whites, this combination of factors results in the concentration of poverty in (often contiguous) urban neighborhoods. Residential separation by social class within each race further compounds the problem of poor quality of neighborhoods for many urban blacks (Massey and Denton, 1993). However, the very existence of substantial black middle-class neighborhoods was questioned in B. Landry's account (1987) of the growth of the black middle class, in which discrimination and black–white segregation are persistent themes. At best, the black middle class could hope to share neighborhoods with skilled and unskilled working class blacks, while only the white middle class had "succeeded in controlling its environment to a large degree" (Landry, 1987).

The importance of neighborhood, beyond social class, in comparing the quality of life for urban blacks and whites can be seen in studies of Philadelphia. In 1980, within specific income levels, higher proportions of blacks than whites lived in neighborhoods with conditions that would be regarded as poorer quality or associated with "underclass" behavior. One component of many definitions of the underclass areas is the high proportion of all births that occur among unwed mothers (Table 1-1). Also, except for the lowest income group, the median value of housing in Philadelphia was lower for blacks than whites. A similar pattern was found for the proportion of students scoring lower than the 15th percentile in SAT scores at the local high school (not shown in Table 1-1). Children from higher income black families were likely to attend a public school where the percentage of low-scoring students was three times greater than at the schools attended by higher income white students (Massey and Denton, 1993). The limitations of using social class alone in the study of black–white differences in quality of life and health should be apparent.

In another highly segregated city (Baltimore), despite the development of an African-American middle class, the concentration of poverty results in great disparities in expenditures per pupil relative to suburban areas. The concentration of poverty and associated family background characteristics (e.g., female-headed households) contribute to the higher high-school dropout rate in the City of Baltimore than in the suburbs (Imbroscio et al., 1995).

These few variables only begin to characterize the potential for neighborhood effects on quality of life and health for blacks. The effect of segregation on the concentration of blacks in high-poverty neighborhoods of metropolitan areas has been referred to by sociologists as "concentration" or "neighborhood" effects. Sociologists have described the various characteristics of urban ghetto life, such as high rates of births to unwed mothers, poor access to goods and services, high rates of exposure to various stresses and violent crime, and a high cost of living (despite high poverty rates) (Chapter 3). These and other factors

Table 1-1. Characteristics of neighborhoods inhabited by blacks and whites of different income levels in Philadelphia, 1980

| | Household income | | | | | | | | |
| | Poor | | | Middle | | | Affluent | | |
Characteristic	White	Black	Black/White	White	Black	Black/White	White	Black	Black/White
Births to unwed mothers (percent)	40.7	37.6	0.9	10.3	25.8	2.5	1.9	16.7	8.8
Median value of homes (thousands of $)	19.4	27.1	1.4	38.0	29.5	0.8	56.6	31.9	0.6

Modified from Massey and Denton (1993, p. 152).

could affect the health status of blacks, as considered in this book. The ultimate causes of high poverty rates in inner cities, and the associated social problems (Fig. 1-1), are under debate, but "structural" factors and "neighborhood" effects are emphasized (Chapter 3). While most poor people, including those regarded as exhibiting "deviant" or socially undesirable behavior are white, the concentration of poverty in certain predominantly minority areas, with their associated "social pathology," gives greater visibility and significance to these behaviors among minorities in a racist society.

The "perinatal paradox" (Kliegman, 1995) refers to the juxtaposition of high-quality medical technology and perinatal care in America with infant mortality rates that are unfavorable relative to many other developed countries (due in part to persistently higher infant mortality rates among blacks than whites). Sophisticated neonatal intensive care units capable of saving the lives of very small infants in hospitals are located in "social and environmental conditions" that jeopardize the surviving infant's health (Kliegman, 1995). The perinatal paradox is especially striking in inner-city areas with large teaching hospitals, such as the one depicted in P. Chayefsky's Oscar-winning script *The Hospital* (1971). In that drama, advanced medical technology stood poised to handle the violent injuries and late-stage medical problems of the surrounding ghettos where basic primary medical care (including immunizations) was woefully inadequate. More generally, while critics of government programs (such as Head Start) emphasize their limitations in terms of outcomes, no single program can conquer poverty and its effects or "overcome the need for decent housing, jobs to provide a living wage, safe neighborhoods, and positive role models" (Zigler and Styfcom, 1996). These are some of the effects of the concentration of poverty (Fig. 1-1).

"Concentration" or "neighborhood" effects may be important in explaining any variation in the overall health (including death rates) of blacks living in different metropolitan areas. Black–white segregation plays a major role in creating and perpetuating these "concentration" effects.

This book examines the evidence for associations between degree of black–white segregation in large urban areas and mortality rates for all causes of death combined for blacks in these areas. Also studied is variation in black/white ratios of death rates for specific age groups among different urban areas. In these analyses, an overall summary measure of social class for blacks in each area is often used, such as the black poverty rate or median household income for all blacks in the area (as published in reports from the U.S. Bureau of the Census). Measures of segregation and black poverty rates are correlated, in a statistical sense, as indicated by the connecting line in Figure 1-1. Therefore, geographic variation in black mortality rates may appear to be correlated with segregation if the distribution of incomes differs for blacks in different areas. This issue is carefully addressed in the analysis and interpretation of variation in death rates for blacks in urban areas.

While the focus is on segregation (due largely to discrimination in housing), it must be recognized that not only blacks in the most highly segregated areas but all blacks are subject to other types of discrimination, well documented by objective studies. This pervasive discrimination may affect the health of blacks through such mechanisms as access to and quality of medical care and psycho-physiological processes. This more direct pathway from discrimination (in its broadest sense) to the health of blacks is indicated in Figure 1-1. While discrimination is the ultimate cause of segregation and the concentration of blacks in high-poverty areas, the relationships between everyday experiences with discrimination and degree of segregation among black persons are apparently poorly understood.

The framework in Figure 1-1 is limited to mechanisms affecting the health of blacks, although death rates for blacks also will be compared with those for whites in large metropolitan areas. White racism, including various types of discriminatory behavior with regard to blacks, could have an impact on the mental and physical health of individual whites. This issue is not addressed in this book, which concentrates on understanding variations in death rates for blacks in large metropolitan areas.

The studies described in this book may be considered as part of the "epidemiology of American apartheid" or the study of the associations between black–white segregation and the health of African Americans. This field could be regarded as an extension of "socioeconomic epidemiology" as introduced by Kitagawa and Hauser (1973). Because discrimination in housing is only one form of discrimination, and other types also could affect the health of all blacks (wherever they live), the "epidemiology of American apartheid" may be considered part of the broader study of the "epidemiology of discrimination and racism."

Some discussion of definitions and issues related to "race" and segregation (Chapter 2) is needed in considering the epidemiology of American apartheid. Chapter 3 deals with the causes and consequences of the concentration of blacks in high-poverty neighborhoods within large metropolitan areas, and with the "concentration" or "neighborhood" effects on quality of life for blacks mentioned earlier.

Chapter 4 considers the evidence for black–white differences in mortality rates in relation to social class, or "socioeconomic epidemiology," and introduces the idea of the epidemiology of American apartheid by drawing analogies with South Africa and (in an extension of socioeconomic epidemiology) by showing the range of variations in black mortality rates among urban areas that might be associated with variation in black poverty rates and in the level of black–white segregation. This is followed by ecologic analyses of variation across large metropolitan areas in death rates for blacks (or black/white ratios of rates), using both social class indicators and degree of segregation for each metropolitan area as independent variables ("predictors") in statistical models of black mortality rates by metropolitan area (Chapter 5). The term *ecologic* refers to studies involving data on social class and segregation for populations in specific metropolitan areas rather than information on the actual histories of individuals with regard to social class and residential segregation in relation to their health and survival.

The limitations of ecologic studies and the interpretation of the findings of these studies are addressed in Chapter 6. The final chapter (Chapter 7) considers some potential implications of the high death rates of blacks found in certain large, hypersegregated metropolitan areas with regard to social and (mainly) health policies. The emphasis is on the role of black communities (especially in ghettos) in public health programs.

2

"Social Race" and Black–White Segregation

Returning to the conceptual framework in Figure 1-1, racial prejudice underlies the discriminatory behavior practiced by whites against blacks. The persistence of segregation is based in part on these attitudes and behaviors, although human attitudes are often not consistent with behavior. Black skin color and (ultimate) ancestry in the African homeland (mainly western Africa) are social markers of African Americans that trigger prejudicial attitudes and discriminatory behavior among whites. White attitudes about the "quality" of neighborhoods, and inceasing emigration, as the proportion of blacks rises are very instructive in this regard.

As noted in Chapter 1, and elaborated later (Chapter 3), the combination of persistent segregation and the perpetuation of high poverty rates in the black population results in the concentration of urban blacks in high-poverty areas. Furthermore, social class stratification within black groups, related to some degree to skin color, also contributes (to a lesser extent) to this concentration of poverty (Massey and Denton, 1993).

Moreover, sociologists and anthropologists have shown that within the black community an association between darker skin color and lower social class (or social status), especially among women, has persisted, (Keith and Herring, 1991; Dressler, 1993). Thus, upward social mobility for blacks continues to be associated with "whiteness" in skin color, as well as with adoption of white values and lifestyle, despite the emergence of black pride and cultural awareness in recent decades. The social relevance of skin color is dramatized by the "bleaching syndrome" or the attempt to overcome the obstacles to assimilation related to the "stigma" of dark skin color within Hispanic populations by the use of "beauty" creams and folk preparations to lighten the color of the skin (Hall, 1994). In *The Fact of Blackness*, Fanon (1992; originally published in French in 1952) wrote of the search for a serum for "denegrification" to "throw off the burden of that corporal malediction" of blackness as viewed by the white majority and incorporated by some blacks in the desire for integration.

13

Hacker (1995) was convinced that "no white American" would consider changing places "with even the most successful black American" because of the loss of "status." In an experiment (undoubtedly unique), a white novelist (Griffin, 1976; originally published in 1960) darkened his skin by medical treatments and confronted the world of pre-civil-rights-era segregation in the South. In *Black Like Me*, Griffin concluded that if whites were placed in ghettos, deprived of educational advantages, and had to "struggle hard to fulfil [their] instinct for self-respect," they would "after a time assume the same characteristics" attached to blacks by some whites." Although this was written several decades ago, the message is still appropriate.

Individuals perceived as "black" based on skin color (and presumed African ancestry) are subject to discrimination in housing. This discrimination and an increase in out-migration of whites from neighborhoods as larger numbers of blacks arrive are the major explanations for black–white segregation. Prejudicial attitudes and discriminatory behavior may be due, in part, to misunderstandings about the significance of "race" (in a biological sense), as well as vague racist ideas (transmitted across generations) about the cultural superiority of "white" or "European" groups.

Definition and Uses of "Social Race"

"Race" and Black "Social Race"

"Race" is often used in a sociopolitical context or by the media without definition and seemingly without recognition of a need for definition, as if the meaning of the term were generally understood. In fact, common usage is undoubtedly riddled with misunderstanding. This also occurs in the scientific and medical literature, where "race" is sometimes used to define groups exclusively on the basis of social and/or cultural differences (as used in sociology) or as a proxy (substitute) variable for social class. However, the term is also used in an ill-defined manner to suggest some biological or genetic distinction.

Many anthropologists and sociologists, especially since the work of M.F. Ashley Montagu (1941), have abandoned "race" in favor of "ethnic group," a term that emphasizes (or is totally restricted to) social and cultural differences between population groups. However, "race" is also used by sociologists strictly with regard to its social significance because genetic differences are regarded as trivial and, in any event, rarely measured in actual studies of health status (Dressler, 1993). In *Preventing Prejudice* (Ponterotto and Pedersen, 1993), for example, the term "race" was said to have "no biological consequences," whereas people's beliefs about race had "profound social consequences." Few would debate the conclusion about social consequences, and "race" is used by sociologists studying trends in groups relations, prejudice and discrimination, and residential segregation.

Realization by scientists that "race" has very limited genetic significance has been a slow process. The term "race" was originally devised as "biological race" during the eighteenth and nineteenth centuries, when biological differences between populations were believed to be great. In *An American Dilemma* (1944) G. Myrdal (1898–1987) recognized the fact that arbitrary social conventions were used to define "racial" groups, based on the pioneering work of the anthropologist F. Boas (1858–1942). In addressing the question, "What is Race" in 1925, Boas wrote that "the variability of the family lines constituting each race will be found so great that . . . we have no right to speak of racial hereditary traits" (in Boas, 1969). This view has been supported abundantly by subsequent research.

Recent research has involved examination of the genetic material (DNA) itself. Restriction enzymes, which "cut" the DNA at specific regions, began to be used to identify restriction fragment length polymorphisms (RFLPs)— differences in the lengths of DNA fragments that result from digestion by specific enzymes. The RFLP method, popularized by media coverage of criminal investigations, is aimed at sites in the human DNA that differ in length due to the presence of varying numbers of "tandemly repeating" units (VNTR). In one study, a panel of 257 RFLP nuclear gene loci was selected because of heterozygosity, or the occurrence of different forms of a gene at a specific locus. About 90% of the total genetic diversity found occurred *within* four "ethnic" groups (also called "races" by Dean et al., 1994). These groups were labeled, following historical convention, as "Caucasians," "African Americans," "American Indians" (Cheyenne from Clinton, Oklahoma), and "Asians" (Chinese residents of Taiwan).

The 90% figure was consistent with earlier estimates (about 85%–90%) based on studies of gene products (that is, blood groups and biochemical markers) rather than analysis of the genes themselves. Obviously, this leaves little room for genetic differences *between* races to play a role in explaining racial differences in disease or risk factors for disease (Polednak, 1989) or in any characteristic.

Unfortunately, even the demonstration of the ultimate kinship of all human populations and the probable African origins of all modern peoples are unlikely to affect race prejudice greatly. Misconceptions about "primitive" African populations that developed during the period of colonialism played an important role in the development of race concepts and have a persistent role in shaping white attitudes (Hacker, 1995). As with any other term, "race" is not inherently evil, but can be used for both humane and inhumane purposes. The danger of overemphasizing small genetic differences between "races," especially with regard to differences in susceptibility to diseases (Jones et al., 1991), is more important than the argument that such genetic differentiation between major groups should not be totally overlooked in medicine and public health (Polednak, 1989). The small genetic differences found between populations can be considered as encompassed by the definition of "ethnic group" or ancestry, without the need for racial groupings (Crews and Bindon, 1991; Cooper, 1994) or "race."

For those who accept "biological race" as a population concept divorced from typological thinking, the frequencies of various genetic "markers" are used in a statistical sense to estimate "distances" between populations. For example, recent work on mitochondrial DNA (located in the cytoplasm rather than the nucleus) has led to recognition of a group of "African" markers in Senegal and other countries of West Africa. The division into "races" is still an arbitrary exercise of convenience for simplifying a complex situation due to a long evolutionary history of population movements across geographic barriers (including continents). Just as dark skin color is not exclusively "African," hemoglobin S (responsible for sickle cell trait and sickle cell disease) is not restricted to a single continent. The rarity of the most common gene mutation responsible for cystic fibrosis in Africa, in comparison with Europe, is part of a geographic gradient (called a "cline" by biologists). For convenience, "West African" population groups can be combined on the basis of some degree of similarity in genetic structure and some common cultural themes. Historically, West African populations provided the "African" component of the majority of the admixed "African-American" group, whether called a race or an ethnic group.

Retaining "race," with the potential for overemphasis of biological and genetic differences between human populations, may contribute to racial prejudice and to overemphasis of the importance of black–white "biological" or genetic differences in explaining disease patterns (Jones et al., 1991). On the other hand, use of "ethnic group" alone may obscure the special significance of dark skin color (and African ancestry) as a social marker (Harrison, 1994, 1995).

Social definitions of race often diverge from any contemporaneous scientific assessment based on actual ancestry. The "one drop rule," or the idea that any amount of African ancestry defined a person as "black" socially, is a striking example of the predominant role of social factors in the definition of "race" (Davis, 1991). The "race" of persons with mixed ancestry has been defined by society and not by themselves (Root, 1992). Noteworthy also has been the attempt to force Puerto Rican Hispanics to select "white" or "black" as a "racial" label, despite the sociocultural inappropriateness of such labels for many (although not all) of these individuals. In the U.S. census, many Hispanics (about 40%) chose "other" race rather than "white" or "black."

In conclusion, social race, as defined by an individual or by society regardless of an individual's own perception, is useful in a discussion of black–white residential segregation. In this book, "black" or "African American" (although "West African American" might be more appropriate) can be used to indicate a heterogeneous population called a "social race."

African-American "race": heterogeneous and multidimensional
Like the African-American population, the black population of Haiti is derived from West Africa (Basu et al., 1976). However, this ancestral aspect is overshadowed by sociocultural factors such as the greater value of "blackness" in the Caribbean and South America than in the United States (Harrison, 1995). Recent immigration from the Caribbean and Central and South America to the United States has resulted in increased ethnic heterogeneity in the "African-American" population. The "Afro-Latino" group is itself diverse in terms of language and ancestry (Bryce-Laporte, 1993).

The need to consider this sociocultural diversity has only recently begun to be appreciated in medicine and public health (Jackson, 1993; Jones et al., 1991), as well as in the social and political sciences (Bryce-Laporte, 1993). For example, better maternal prenatal profiles and greater fetal intrauterine growth were found for foreign-born than U.S.-born black women seen at Boston City Hospital (Cabral et al., 1990). A study of incidence rates of breast and uterine cervix cancers in Caribbean immigrant versus U.S.-born black women in Brooklyn, NY, showed higher rates of cervical cancer for Haitian women, which could reflect low cancer screening rates in Haiti, as well as the United States (Fruchter et al., 1990). England and Wales also have diverse black populations, including immigrants from West Africa, East Africa, and the Caribbean. These populations exhibit complex patterns of cancer mortality rates (Grulich et al., 1992).

African Americans are also genetically diverse as measured in individuals and in populations defined by geographic criteria. The degree of "admixture" or gene flow between racial groups can be estimated by various methods (Chakraborty, 1986). Extensive and accurate (error-free) genealogies that cover multiple generations are rarely available. Instead, data on skin color, a complex and poorly understood genetic marker, have been used, along with frequencies of certain blood groups and serum proteins. The number of genetic "markers" that can be used to distinguish populations in terms of their relative frequencies has grown with technological advances.

Human leukocyte antigens (HLA), originally discovered on white blood cells, differ in frequency across racial and ethnic groups. These antigens are relevant not only to tissue matching for organ transplantation but also to disease susceptibility, especially for diseases involving dysfunction of the immune system. The importance of HLA tissue typing is mentioned later with regard to kidney transplants in blacks and whites (Chapter 6). HLA antigens and other genetic markers, involving, for example, the familiar Rh (Rhesus) and the less-familiar Duffy blood groups, have been used to estimate the amount of gene flow or intermixture between populations defined as "African" and "European." Using data on 15 polymorphic loci that encode for proteins, the proportion of white genes in U.S. blacks living in the greater Pittsburgh metropolitan area was estimated at 25% (Chakraborty et al., 1992). Included were 18 "unique" variants that occur only in blacks and 5 variants restricted to whites. Individuals as well as groups can be characterized by their level of admixture, using a variable number of genetic markers.

The multidimensional nature of "race" or "ethnic group" is illustrated by considering the higher prevalence of hypertension in African Americans than in whites. Hypertension is commonly defined (in the U.S. National Health Survey) as "elevated" blood pressure (140 + mmHg systolic or 90 + mmHg diastolic) or "definite hypertension" (165 + systolic and/or 95 + diastolic and/or the use of antihypertensive medications).

A 1957 report, "An Epidemiologic Study of Blood Pressure Levels in a Biracial Community in the Southern United States," reprinted in 1995 (Comstock, 1995) with an accompanying commentary (Kuller, 1995), concluded that the observed black–white differences in adult blood pressures were not necessarily "racial" (i.e., genetic) in character. Interestingly, historically higher blood pressure levels in rural than urban American blacks, based on studies of rural blacks done prior to the civil rights era, suggested that "racist psychosocial stress" in rural areas might have been involved (Wilson et al., 1991). Differing levels of black–white genetic admixture by urban–rural residence (i.e., the North vs. the South) could not be ruled out.

Studies of racial admixture, now included in genetic epidemiology, could be potentially useful in evaluating the issue of genetic factors in explaining racial differences in disease (Khoury and Beaty, 1994). The results of studies using skin color as an index of black–white admixture have been inconsistent (Gleiberman et al., 1995). However, skin color not only is an indicator of admixture but also is associated with social status (especially for women) (Keith and Herring, 1991). In a study in three U.S. cities, the association between darker skin color and blood pressure in black adults was limited to the lower social classes (Klag et al., 1991). This suggests that environmental factors associated with lower social class may be crucial whether or not a susceptible genotype (Parmer et al., 1994) is more common among African populations.

One mechanism in the development of hypertension is vasoconstriction (reduction in the diameter of blood vessels) related to the hormones epinephrine (also called adrenaline) and norepinephrine (noradrenaline), which are released from sympathetic nerves. A variety of black–white differences in vasoconstriction in response to stresses have been documented (Sherwood et al., 1995). This could be responsible for a cascade of effects, including those involving the activity of insulin and the internal balance between sodium and potassium levels. The details of these putative mechanisms need not concern us here. The main point is that stresses and responses to stress that differ between blacks and whites could be important (Chapter 6).

Self-reported race and acculturation
The classification of individuals should be by self-report (from multiple choice items) and not based on perceptions of others as the "principal criterion" (Hahn and Stroup, 1994). Indeed, this is a common (though not universal) practice.

Objective rating scales for ethnic identification, based on respondents' perceptions and attitudes, have been developed. For blacks, black racial identity or consciousness scales consist of as many as 42, 50, and 65 items (Ponterotto and Pedersen, 1993). In research studies, much shorter scales have been used. One scale includes "historical allegiance" to the value of Africans as creators of civilization, the importance of the culture of one's ancestors in daily life, and (perhaps most arguably) the specific term used for ethnic identity (with "African" being stronger than "African American," "black" or "Negro") (Scribner et al., 1995). Historically, many terms have been used (Stuckey, 1987).

The 1930s witnessed a major struggle for black physicians to convince the *Journal of the American Medical Association* to capitalize "Negro" in order to "elicit some respect from white physicians" (Charatz-Litt, 1992). This practice had also been advocated by W.E.B. Du Bois, although there was disagreement about the use of "Negro" (a label derived from whites and associated with slavery, but not considered derogatory by all blacks) (Stuckey, 1987). While white physicians published little work about black health issues for several decades (Charatz-Litt, 1992), black–white differences in disease and risk factors have received increasing attention in the medical literature, although the term "race" (especially for blacks) has been misused (Osborne and Feit, 1992).

Disregarding the issue of labels, racial or ethnic identification scales for blacks also could be considered as elements of acculturation, the process of influencing cultural patterns (e.g., language, diet, religion, music, and art) that occurs when two or more groups come into contact. Although early definitions of acculturation recognized a two-way process of mutual influencing, the loss of language and other cultural elements by the migrant or minority group is often emphasized. In one anthropological scheme, "assimilation, " or the melding of cultural identity into the mainstream culture, is distinct from "integration," which refers to the adoption of certain mainstream values or behaviors, but with the retention of some original elements of one's ancestral culture. "Marginalization" is the rejection of both cultures (Berry et al., 1987; Richman et al., 1987), resembling the ideas of "subculture" and "counterculture" used by sociologists (Chapter 3).

Items used in acculturation scales for Hispanics, such as language preference and proficiency (English vs. Spanish) and birthplace of parents and grandparents, seem less relevant to most blacks, except for birthplace of parents among recent immigrants. However, inner-city blacks exhibit distinctive English language patterns or a vernacular (Attinasi, 1994; Massey and Denton, 1993), including the use of abbreviated forms of common words. Acculturation measures in Hispanics include items related to the "degree of pride" in Hispanic and Latino heritage and the ethnicity of one's closest friends (Cuellar et al., 1980; Feliz-Ortiz et al., 1994; Hazuda et al., 1988), which resemble (in some ways) the ethnic identity scales developed for blacks (Jackson, 1992). These scales have been used in a few studies of health and mortality in blacks (Chapter 6).

The use of "race" in censuses and vital records
In 1954, Allport noted that children should "learn the confusion that occurs between genetic and social definitions of race" and that a "caste" definition of black and white race obscures the "biological fact" that some blacks are "racially as much" white as black (See Allport, 1969). Since 1989, the National Center for Health Statistics has considered infants of "mixed" (black and white) race to be "black" if the mother is black. Since American blacks are admixed with whites, the offspring of such "mixed" parents would be more "white" than "black" in a biological sense. This practice may be regarded as a vestige of the "one-drop rule" (Davis, 1991).

There is increasing interest in the issue of separate recognition of "mixed race" persons, including the need for modification of Bureau of the Census questionnaires to permit individuals to choose "mixed" categories (Hunt, 1993) or multiple categories (Root, 1992), including multiple "ancestral" backgrounds, such as "West African." The implications of these proposals for epidemiology, as well as political repercussions, require further discussion (Cooper, 1994).

An exception to the predominance of self-reported "race" has been the use of "race" as defined by perceptions of hospital clerks working with hospital discharge databases in many states (including New York and California). This is reportedly due to a reluctance to ask patients direct questions (sometimes regarded as sensitive) (Blustein, 1994). Unfortunately, due to such practices the reliability and repeatability of racial classification of the same individual at two different hospitals is poor. On death certificates, certifiers (with unknown frequency) make subjective assessments of race and ethnicity without asking the next of kin, leading to discrepancies in race and ethnicity codes on birth and death records of the same individual. However, such inconsistency has been lower for black (4%) than for Hispanic (30%) and American Indian (47%) and certain other groups of infants (Hahn et al., 1992).

Historically, there have been shifts in opinion in the United States as to the desirability of recording information on race and ethnicity in public or official documents (including health records). However, the absence of adequate information on racial and ethnic differences in disease and mortality is often criticized because the effects of inequities in health care possibly due to discrimination and racism cannot then be examined.

In this book, mortality rates are analyzed for "white" and "black" populations living in different metropolitan areas in the United States. The denominators for these rates are population estimates from the U.S. census, where individuals are asked to declare their "race" (e.g., "white" and "black"). Numerator and death information is from death certificates, where the source of information on race is more uncertain. Such complexities as degree of admixture, extent of racial intermarriage, and degree of ethnic identification cannot be assessed.

Black–White Intermarriage, Acculturation, and Segregation

The genetic counterpart of the sociocultural process of acculturation is "race mixture" or admixture. This process is influenced by sociocultural factors such as degree of isolation and attitudes about group interaction. Exogamy, or marriage between persons of different racial or ethnic backgrounds, is a major force in acculturation and largely determines the long-term existence of ethnic groups as recognizable entities (Stevens and Swicegood, 1987). Thus, for many Americans, especially those with ancestors from many different ethnic groups, ethnicity has become vague or even meaningless (Steinberg, 1989).

However, the percentage of all U.S. married couples who were mixed (black and white) increased slightly from 0.15% in 1970 to 0.34% in 1980, with a smaller increase by 1990 (0.40% or 211,000 black–white married couples) (U.S. Bureau of the Census, 1994). Among new marriages in 1980, 6,261 involved a black groom and a white bride, while 2,289 involved a white groom and a black bride; corresponding figures for 1987 were 8,447 and 3,289, representing slight increases, but the total number of marriages was more than 1.5

million in each year (National Center for Health Statistics, 1991). Thus, while the temporal increase in the number of black–white married couples has been emphasized by some observers, the proportion of such marriages remains very small.

While the persistence of relatively small numbers of black–white marriages is due largely to attitudes of whites, the rise of "Afrocentrism," black pride and anti-assimilation feelings among some blacks, has also led to opposition to intermarriage. Assimilationist views have the danger of fostering the devaluation of blackness, including characteristics of skin color and hair form, and social hierarchies among blacks may be based on white-influenced perceptions of beauty (Connor, 1995; hooks, 1995; West, 1994). Another factor may be fear of "cultural genocide" and other forms of "genocide" (e.g., with reference to the AIDS epidemic) (Thomas and Quinn, 1991).

White attitudes about interracial marriage in America reflect complex historical, cultural, social, and psychological influences. In *An American Dilemma,* Myrdal (1944) reported the results of a national survey (in 1939) showing that the issue of intermarriage and sexual intercourse between blacks and whites was the first (of six) in importance for whites but last for blacks. Surveys since the 1940s suggest a difference between attitudes about personal versus societal practices regarding interracial dating or marriage. In national surveys from the 1960s to the 1980s (Schuman et al., 1985; Firebaugh and Davis, 1988), approval of black–white intermarriages has been much higher among blacks than whites. Among blacks, approval was 78% in 1983, similar to the 76% figure for 1972; for whites the figures were 40% in 1983 and 27% in 1972. Disagreement with laws prohibiting "racial intermarriage" increased some over time, remaining lower in the South (where less than 50% opposed such laws in 1982).

Key tenets of racist ideologies include the idea that "miscegenation" or racial intermixture results in "lower biological quality." Such beliefs persist despite the contrary evidence from physical anthropologists (Davis, 1991) and genetic epidemiologists (Khoury and Beaty, 1994). Scientific racism and eugenics, including the theory of "hybrid degeneracy" or "unstable genetic constitution," were prevalent in the early twentieth century (Nakashima, 1992). Some whites remain "intractable" with regard to the issue of "race crossings" (Fanon, 1992), which may influence attitudes about racial intermarriage. Fears of the results of racial mixture, along with beliefs in large biological differences between whites and blacks, were commonly expressed in interviews of members of extremist racist groups in America (Ezekiel, 1995).

An emerging area of research in epidemiology is the study of differences among groups defined as "mixed" with regard to the effects of their psychosocial experiences on health. In a study of infants in Illinois in 1982–1983, of a higher rate of low birthweight was found for infants of black mothers and white fathers than among those of white mothers and black fathers (Collins and David, 1993). This finding cannot be easily explained by genetic factors but probably reflects the effects of racism and other psychosocial or psychophysiological factors experienced by black mothers (Chapter 6). In Brazil, recognition of "mulatto(e)s" has persisted (in contrast to the "one-drop rule" in the United States). Cancer rates have been compared among ethnic groups in São Paulo (Bouchardy et al., 1991). The method of classification of the ethnic groups ("blacks," "mulattos," and "whites") was not clear, but self-reporting was apparently not involved. Lower rates for many cancer sites were found in blacks and mulattos relative to whites (Bouchardy et al., 1991). The medical and public health literature, even after the racist works of the nineteenth century (Krieger, 1987), has tended to concentrate on diseases more common in blacks (Osborne and Feit, 1992), perhaps reflecting not only research funding priorities but also subtle (institutional) racism. On the other hand, the targeting of research and of prevention programs to groups at relatively high risk for specific diseases or risk factors has been a tradition in public health.

Relative to U.S. whites and blacks, the degree of segregation among whites, blacks, and mulattoes (browns) in Brazil is considerably lower and intermarriage more common (especially in the lower classes) (Telles, 1992). The pattern of increasing racial intermarriage and recognition of mixed races in Brazil and other countries such as Colombia was once thought to be the wave of the future in America (Jaynes and Williams, 1989). However, the small increases in the numbers of black–white intermarriages and out-of-wedlock births (Davis, 1991) have paralleled the slow decline in black–white residential segregation (as discussed in the next section).

Black–White Segregation in America

Definitions and Trends

Interviewing virtually all 10,000 blacks in the seventh Ward of Philadelphia in 1896, which contained about one-fourth of all blacks in the city, Du Bois (1973; originally published in 1899) described the plight of blacks, many recently arrived from the South, who found a life that was "hard, noisy and deadly" (Lewis, 1993). In a sense, these migrants stood out "conspicuously" by their skin and culture, yet their social and economic problems were largely ignored (and in this sense they were invisible). Blacks were being banned from their traditional jobs in catering and barbering, as well as from craft and industrial unions dominated by European immigrants. World Wars I and II, with an interruption during the Depression, brought job opportunities in the industrial North and Midwest, but also increased competition between a growing black minority and the white populations of these areas. Many northern cities, such as Cleveland and Milwaukee, showed large increases in black–white segregation starting around 1910–1920, and by 1940 black–white residential segregation was entrenched as an institution. The history of residential segregation has been described in detail elsewhere (e.g., Farley and Frey, 1992, 1994; Fuchs, 1990; Lieberson, 1980; Massey and Denton, 1987, 1993). However, some discussion of definitions and time trends will help clarify analyses of regional patterns in black mortality rates (Chapters 5 and 6).

Definition of metropolitan statistical areas
Residential segregation has been measured in a large number of urban areas based on data from decennial censuses. Metropolitan statistical areas (MSAs), or standard metropolitan statistical areas (SMSAs) in the earlier literature, are defined by the Federal Office of Management and Budget (OMB). Revised definitions for 1993 (OMB Bulletin No. 93-05) included 253 MSAs and 62 primary MSAs (PMSAs). The 62 PMSAs are part of 19 larger units called consolidated MSAs, which are too large to be useful for the present purposes. MSAs and PMSAs consist of a large population nucleus or center (usually a central city) and adjacent communities that are associated economically and socially with the nucleus. The subunits of MSAs and PMSAs are counties, except in New England, where cities or towns are used. MSAs and PMSAs vary greatly in population size, but the total area must reach 100,000 (or 75,000 in New England).

Measurement of the "segregation index"
The index of residential segregation for each MSA and PMSA used in this book is the "index of residential dissimilarity" or D_{xy} (often written simply as "D"), well-known to sociologists. D is equal to half the sum (among all "n" census tracts or smaller subunits of an MSA) of the absolute values of $[(x_i/X) - (y_i/Y)]$, where x_i and y_i are the populations of each racial-ethnic group (e.g., "blacks" and "Anglos" [non-Hispanic whites]) within a given tract (i), and X and Y are the total populations for each race in the MSA (Lieberson, 1980). Thus, the index indicates the degree of unevenness in the residential distribution of minority and majority groups across all census tracts within an urban area.

Theoretically, D may vary from 0.00 to 1.00, but D is often multiplied by 100 (as by Farley and Frey, 1992, 1994). D is an indication of the proportion of blacks who would have to move in order to achieve an even distribution of blacks or the absence of segregation (Massey and Denton, 1993). D is the same for each of the two ethnic groups and is unaffected by the *numbers* in each group, except for the effect that small numbers of persons have on sampling errors in the estimation of D.

D should be distinguished from measures of the potential for contact or "interaction" between members of two racial or ethnic groups within census tracts of urban areas, or the isolation of each group, which consider the *numbers* of residents of each ethnic group as well as their spatial distribution. These measures (unlike D) can be calculated for each ethnic group (x and y). As D increases, the isolation index for blacks tends to increase and the degree of potential contact between the two groups decreases. This book is less concerned with the interaction potential between blacks and Anglos than with the pattern of spatial segregation, which may be related to quality of life factors that could influence mortality rates for blacks.

In the first example in Table 2-1 (from Lieberson, 1980), D is 0.5 times the sum of the absolute values of $[(30/100) - (370/1,000)] + [(10/100) - (290/1,000)] + [(0/100) - 300/1,000)] + [(60/100) - (40/1000)]$, or 0.5 times 1.12 or 0.56. In the second example in Table 2-1, the data were not changed for Anglos but the distribution of blacks was modified so that all blacks in the city or MSA live in one subarea or census tract. D is 0.96.

The value of D does not reach 1.00 (or 100% segregation) in the second example, because a few whites live in the subarea where all blacks live, If there were no whites in this all-black subarea, the value of D would be 1.00 (or 100% segregation). In the first example in Table 2-1, while D is almost at its maximum attainable value of 1.0, there is still some potential for contact between blacks and Anglos within one census tract (or whatever type of subunit is involved). In contrast, if the proportion of blacks living in each subarea or census tract were the same as the proportion of blacks in the entire population of the MSA, the value of D would be zero (0%). In this situation, no black persons would have to move to achieve an even distribution of blacks among the subareas.

Indexes of residential segregation (D), calculated by using block groups (units smaller than census tracts), are shown in Table 2-2 for the 38 MSAs that had a total population of more than 1 million in 1980. The use of census block groups (Farley and Frey, 1992, 1994) results in larger and more accurate segregation indexes for neighborhoods than those obtained by using the larger census tract units. The average population of a census tract is around 4,000 (with much variation across tracts), whereas block groups averaged about 900 in 1980 and 560 in 1990. With reference to the formula cited earlier, D is often multiplied by 100. The highest segregation index in 1990 was 90 (for Chicago). Several other MSAs had high indexes, mainly in the East and Midwest (for example, Detroit at 89 in both 1980 and 1990). These indexes are very close to the theoretical maximum of 100. The lowest segregation index was 43 (for Anaheim–Santa Ana, CA), and only one other MSA had had an index less than 50. Thus, the lowest indexes are far from the theoretical minimum. However, there is some variation in the degree of black–white segregation (Table 2-2). This variation is useful in the analyses of mortality rates by MSA (Chapter 5).

Table 2-1. Illustration of calculation of an index of residential segregation (D) for metropolitan statistical areas (MSAs)

Census	Example 1				Example 2			
Tract (i)	Blacks (x)	Anglos (y)	Total	Percent black	Black (x)	Anglos (y)	Total	Percent black
1	30	370	400	0.075	0	370	370	0.000
2	10	290	300	0.033	0	290	290	0.000
3	0	300	300	0.000	0	300	300	0.000
4	60	40	100	0.600	100	40	140	0.700
Total	100 (X)	1,000 (Y)	1,100	0.091	100 (X)	1,000 (Y)	1,100	0.091
			D = 0.56				D = 0.96	

Example 1 is after Lieberson (1980).
In this table, "x" and "y" are the black and Anglo populations in each census tract, and "X" and "Y" are the total black and Anglo populations for the entire MSA (all tracts combined) (see text for formula for calculating "D").

Table 2-2. Change in segregation index in 38 MSAs from 1980 to 1990

MSA*	Segregation Index		Percent change
	1980	1990	
Anaheim	47	43	−0.09
Atlanta	79	73	−0.08
Baltimore	78	75	−0.04
Boston	76	70	−0.08
Buffalo	84	84	0.0†
Chicago	91	87	−0.04
Cincinnati	82	80	−0.02
Cleveland	89	86	−0.03
Columbus	76	71	−0.07
Dallas	81	66	−0.19
Denver	70	66	−0.06
Detroit	89	89	0.0†
Fort Lauderdale	86	73	−0.15
Houston	78	69	−0.12
Indianapolis	83	80	−0.04
Kansas City	81	76	−0.06
Los Angeles	80	71	−0.11
Miami	81	75	−0.07
Milwaukee	85	84	−0.01
Minneapolis	70	65	−0.07
Nassau and Suffolk Counties, NY	80	79	−0.01
New Orleans	76	74	−0.03
New York, NY	78	78	0.0†
Newark	84	83	−0.01
Philadelphia	83	82	−0.01
Phoenix	62	51	−0.18
Pittsburgh	75	75	0.0†
Portland, OR	73	68	−0.07
Riverside	58	49	−0.16
Sacramento	60	58	−0.03
St. Louis	85	81	−0.05
San Antonio	65	57	−0.12
San Diego	63	59	−0.06
San Francisco	68	65	−0.04
San Jose	48	45	−0.06
Seattle	69	60	−0.13
Tampa	82	74	−0.10
Washington, DC	71	68	−0.04

Data are from Farley and Frey (1994a, b).

* Names are abbreviated.

† No change.

Time trends in segregation in large MSAs

For 38 MSAs listed in Table 2-2 used in analyses of mortality rates (Chapter 5), the average index of black–white segregation declined from 75 in 1980 to 71 in 1990. In many large metropolitan areas of the northeastern and north central or midwestern United States, residential segregation of blacks from Anglos has not decreased in recent decades (Table 2-2), even in middle-class areas (Massey and Denton, 1993). If segregation remains constant, any increase in the (already high) overall poverty rate for blacks in an MSA will accentuate the concentration of poverty in segregated, predominantly black areas within the MSA. Temporal increases in black poverty rates have occurred in recent decades in some MSAs in the North and Midwest (Massey and Denton, 1993), and these trends have implications for the concentration of poverty in "ghettos" (as discussed in Chapter 3).

Massey and Denton's analysis of segregation trends (1993) focused on 30 large MSAs that included a large proportion of the country's black population. For 18 metropolitan areas in the North combined, the average degree of segregation declined very slightly from 1970 to 1990. For some of the most highly segregated areas, such as the metropolitan areas of Gary, IN, and Detroit, MI (Fig. 2-1), there was no decline. For 12 metropolitan areas in the South, the average segregation index declined somewhat more than in the North, but trends for individual areas varied. The Norfolk, VA, area had the lowest index of these 30 areas in 1990, but the value was still 50 using census tracts (Fig. 2-1)

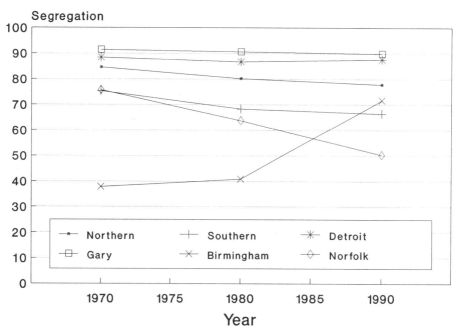

Figure 2-1. Trend in the degree of black–white residential segregation in the United States.

and 57, using census-block data (Farley and Frey, 1992). Norfolk was the only area among the 30 that had a segregation index less than 60%, or a level considered not "high" by Massey and Denton (1993).

However, the apparent increase in segregation in Birmingham in Figure 2-1 is based on the use of census tracts as subunits in calculating the segregation index by MSA. Using census-block groups (i.e., subdivisions of census tracts), Farley and Frey (1992) reported an index of 80 for Birmingham in 1980. While Farley and Frey (1992) did not report segregation indexes for 1970 or earlier years, Massey and Denton (1993) showed that, using census blocks as units, the segregation index for Birmingham actually declined slightly from 93 in 1960 and 92 in 1970 to 79 in 1990. In his "Letter from a Birmingham Jail" in 1963, Martin Luther King Jr. referred to Birmingham as "probably the most thoroughly segregated city in the United States" (Washington, 1992) with regard to the attitudes of whites in Birmingham during the 1960s.

The distinctive history of blacks is manifested (and perpetuated) by the residential segregation of blacks from whites (i.e,. Anglos or non-Hispanic whites), which continues to be much higher than that between Anglos and either Hispanics or Asians (Massey and Denton, 1987, 1993). Ethnic "enclaves" have been transitional for many ethnic groups as social mobility and spatial mobilty increased across the generations, but the persistence of urban ghettos represents a different phenomenon (Lieberson, 1980; Massey and Denton, 1993).

W.E.B. Du Bois (around 1940) predicted that segregation would last for generations to come (Stuckey, 1987). In effect, "basic mobility" for blacks is still largely, as described by King, "from a larger ghetto to a smaller one" (Washington, 1992). In some smaller cities, with small proportions of blacks, segregation has shown an appreciable temporal decline. Among all 318 MSAs, the number that can be classified as "moderately" segregated (D less than 55) increased from 29 in 1980 to 68 in 1990; included were MSAs with large retirement communities, with larger numbers of middle-class blacks (e.g., Riverside, CA) or improving economic conditions for blacks, and areas with new housing construction (e.g., San Jose and Anaheim–Santa Ana, CA) (Farley and Frey, 1992, 1994). Some sociologists have regarded these minor declines in segregation as a sign of progress and a hope for the future (Farley and Frey, 1992, 1994). However, other sociologists have noted that the pace is so slow that many decades are required to achieve significant integration of the entire black population (Massey and Denton, 1993).

Prejudice versus discrimination

The prevalence of expressed antiblack prejudice and segregationist attitudes has been declining in surveys in the United States, especially in the South (Schuman et al., 1985; Firebaugh and Davis, 1998). Since the groundbreaking work of Myrdal's team in *An American Dilemma* (1944), which included a survey for *Fortune* magazine conducted by the Roper Center for Public Opinion Research in 1939, major sources of data on attitudes of whites and blacks have included surveys by the National Opinion Research Center at the University of Chicago (starting in 1942), the Institute for Social Research at the University of

Michigan, and the Gallup and Harris organizations (as compiled by Schuman et al., 1985). Large numbers of whites no longer attempt to justify segregation in principle, although change with regard to racial intermarriage has been less striking (as discussed earlier in this chapter). Questions on principles dealt with school integration, residential integration, integration of public transportation, and job discrimination. Most striking was the trend toward acceptance of school integration among whites, reaching 90% by 1982. However, the proportion of white respondents favoring "desegregation" peaked around 1970 and declined thereafter, while the proportion favoring "something in between" rose after 1970.

Despite the trends suggesting declines in prejudicial attitudes among whites, although not always clear cut, the decline in black–white segregation in the post-civil rights era has been slow. "Audit" studies use two or more individuals differing in race or ethnicity but matched on all characteristics defined (a priori) as relevant; each person applies for the same job, housing, or specific service, and their experiences are recorded (Fix and Strucyk, 1993). In audit studies by the Urban Institute in Chicago, New York, Los Angeles, and Atlanta, 40%–45% of audits involved less fair treatment of blacks than whites with regard to housing sales (36%–49% for rentals).

Sociological survey research shows that the aversion of whites to living in racially integrated neighborhoods stems from whites associating integration with higher crime rates, deteriorating quality of neighborhoods, and declining property values. Even when these associations were taken into account in experimental studies where hypothetical "vignette" neighborhoods were described to survey respondents, perceived neighborhood "quality" was adversely affected by increasing proportions of blacks (St. John and Bates, 1989). Surveys of "neighborhood preferences" of whites, as in the Detroit Area Survey of 1976, showed that discomfort with, attempts to move out of, or refusal to move into a neighborhood changed as the proportion of blacks increased. A neighborhood about one-third black represented the limit of racial tolerance for the majority of whites. Surveys in other cities have shown similar results (reviewed by Massey and Denton, 1993). Consistent with these surveys, a seemingly inexorable "ghettoization" process occurs, with a change in both racial and socioeconomic composition, once the black population reaches a certain proportion of the total population.

The causes of segregation are discussed at considerable length in Chapter 4 of Massey and Denton's *American Apartheid* (1993). "Group threat" and "group contact" theories are mentioned briefly here. According to group threat theory in sociology and the results of analyses of survey data on prejudice and discrimination in European groups, the greater number of African Americans (vs. Asian Americans) may help to account for the greater prejudice experienced by blacks (Quillian, 1995) and hence for their greater degree of segregation. This view is consistent with the rise of segregation after the migration of blacks from the South to the North and with early descriptions by W.E.B. Du Bois on the exclusion of blacks from labor unions and the usurping of many previously "black" occupations by whites. Lieberson (1980) argued that economic competition between blacks and whites, resulting from increasing black population size, led to a deterioration of the social position of blacks in the North.

Some liberals influenced by Myrdal came to believe that greater contact between the races (especially among school children) would undoubtedly contribute to a reduction in prejudice (Jackson, 1990) and, presumably, in discrimination. The "social contact" theory of reducing prejudice has received some support from the work of Israeli social scientists on the process of integration of (black) Ethiopian Jews into Israeli society, where greater exposure to these "outsiders" was associated with lower "social distance" scores (Goldberg and Kirschenbaum, 1989). In America, opportunities for cross-race interaction influence interracial sociability and friendship, but data from the national High School and Beyond Survey showed that high school students were only about one-sixth as likely to choose a cross-race as a same-race peer as a friend. School organizational characteristics, such as "tracking," appeared to be influential in this process (Firebaugh and Davis, 1988; Hallinan and Williams, 1989; Jaynes and Williams, 1989).

Extreme Segregation: Public Housing Projects

Public housing projects are here discussed briefly because they are considered later with reference to the potential health effects of segregation (Chapter 5) and public health programs in urban black communities (Chapter 7).

"Urban renewal" facilitated the extreme segregation and crowding of blacks into public housing projects or "reservations" in hypersegregated cities such as Chicago and New York (Massey and Denton, 1993). While the construction of public housing projects has reached a virtual standstill (Table 2-3), large numbers of units still exist (i.e., about 1.4 million occupied units in 1988). More than 3.5 million people live in these units, which are administered by about 3,000 public housing authorities, and about 75% of residents are minorities (Williams and Kornblum, 1995).

Variability in quality of life in housing projects has been recognized, although research on this issue appears to be limited. Not all projects may fit the pattern of Chicago's black-occupied Cabrini-Green and Robert Taylor Homes, where a disproportionately large share of Chicago's crimes (murders, assaults, and

Table 2-3. Low-income public housing units (in thousands) in the United States

Year	Total	Occupied	Under construction
1960	593.3	478.2	36.4
1970	1,155.3	893.5	126.8
1980	1,321.1	1,195.6	20.9
1988	1,448.8	1,413.3	9.7

From *Statistical Abstract of the United States, 1994* (U.S. Bureau of the Census, 1994).

rapes), gunshot wounds and firearms confiscations occur (Wilson, 1987). Some of the Midwest's larger segregated public housing projects, such as in St. Louis and (more recently) Chicago, have been "destroyed as unlivable" (Wilson, 1987). On the other hand, four East Harlem, NY, housing projects may provide low-income housing for working low-income, predominantly minority persons (and their families) who would otherwise be homeless (Williams and Kornblum, 1995). These housing projects have been described as "priceless but embattled centers of neighborhood strength and empowerment." Not all projects, at least in East Harlem, provide a high-crime environment deleterious for childhood and adolescent development, due in part to vigorous tenant organizations and their cooperation with project managers. In comparison with the surrounding decaying, higher crime neighborhoods, some East Harlem projects provide relatively safe areas for social support, although demands placed on the resources and "courage" of residents may be "overwhelming."

In comparison with Chicago housing projects (Wilson, 1987), some East Harlem housing projects had higher proportions of working poor, lower proportions of people receiving Aid for Families with Dependent Children (AFDC), and better physical conditions (such as indoor elevators). Critics could argue that the "relative success" of some housing projects in East Harlem may contribute to the maintenance of "patterns of racial and class segregation which public housing fostered" (Williams and Kornblum, 1995).

Conclusion

The salience of dark skin and/or "African" ancestry is shown by the persistence of black–white urban segregation, with the minor progress in recent decades being limited to small metropolitan areas where blacks comprise small proportions of the total populations. Social scientists continue to examine trends in segregation and have attempted to explain its persistence.

Sociologist J. Quadragno (1994) revived Myrdal's "dilemma" thesis in her historical account of the role of racism in the American welfare state, where recognition of the "blemish" of racial segregation on the "American conscience" has been overwhelmed by the desire to maintain white privileges in housing and jobs. In view of the hugely unsuccessful "separate but equal" model, whether espoused by whites or blacks, the reality of segregation and the fact that blacks still often attend black-majority schools has suggested the need for "forceful multicultural education" as part of a larger effort of black communities to understand and attempt to overcome their problems (Glazer, 1993).

According to a proverb in the Yoruba language of West Africa, collected by Sir R. Burton, "He who torments another (only) teaches him to strengthen himself." The "strengthening" of individual self-identification with "race" and cohesion of groups undergoing discrimination and oppression has been described with reference to Jews and blacks (Steinberg, 1989; Henry, 1990). However, the psychosocial toll in blacks of all social classes of dealing with discrimination may be great (Feagin, 1991). Also, the quest for group cohesion or empowerment may promote a reluctance to address the issue of segregation and its effects on quality of social and physical environment (Massey and Denton, 1993). As Allport (1969) observed, until "segregation is weakened, conditions will not exist that permit equal social status contacts in pursuit of common objectives." At the same time, it is understandable that blacks "cannot wait for an end to racist domination" to provide for "sustained well being" (hooks, 1995). Yet hooks does not abandon hope for a "beloved community" (in the words of King) in which "allegiances to special cultural legacies" are not lost.

Understanding the full implications of segregation for the quality of life and health of urban blacks requires considering the importance of the combined effect of high black poverty rates and high levels of segregation in some urban areas. These "concentration" or "neighborhood" effects are discussed in the next chapter.

3

Black Poverty, Segregation, and "Concentration" or "Neighborhood" Effects

The central theme of this book is that the concentration of blacks in high-poverty urban areas, with adverse effects on their quality of life, also may affect their health (Fig. 1-1). The previous chapter addressed segregation as one of the two elements of this combination of factors. This chapter describes features of the distribution of poverty or low income among African-Americans, including temporal changes in black poverty rates in certain urban areas.

The terms *poverty* and *the poor* are generally used not only in an ill-defined colloquial sense but also according to a well-established (albeit highly criticized) offical government definition. The poverty threshold as originally defined by the Social Security Administration in 1964 was based on a determination that families of three or more persons spent (in 1961) one-third of their income on food. Thus, the cost of a nutritionally adequate food plan designed by the Department of Agriculture was multiplied by three, and factors were developed to adjust for differing family sizes. The U.S. Bureau of the Census has provided annual modifications of poverty thresholds, based solely on adjustment for the annual consumer price index (CPI), relative to CPI in 1982–1984. The average thresholds for a family of four persons were $2,973 in 1959, $3,743 in 1969, $7,412 in 1979, $12,674 in 1989, and $14,335 in 1992.

Federal poverty thresholds were intended to indicate an income level, adjusted for family size and age, sufficient for adequate nutrition, not to be an indicator of deprivation or destitution. However, the lack of change in the methodology for calculating poverty thresholds over time has had the effect that such thresholds are now indicative of very low income. The declining relevance of the poverty threshold is due in part to a decline in proportion of income spent on food (vs. housing and other expenses), with a somewhat counterbalancing effect of increases in noncash or "in-kind" public assistance benefits such as food stamps, Medicaid, and housing subsidies.

The immense literature critiquing poverty level definitions is not reviewed here. Population surveys show that public perceptions and attitudes support the conclusion that official poverty thresholds are too low to capture a large segment of the population with incomes inadequate to provide basic necessities or protection from having to make difficult choices between providing adequate food, clothing, or medical care for themselves and their family members (Jencks, 1992). A threshold of 155% of the official poverty line has been proposed to define "self-sufficiency" (Schwarz and Volgy, 1992).

The Bureau of the Census has recognized the limitations of the poverty thresholds and has published data on the proportions of the populations at various fractions or multiples of the threshold. Thus, the ratio of the income of individuals or families to their appropriate poverty threshold is reported (e.g., <0.50, 1.00–1.25, and ≥ 1.75), although most of the detailed tables are limited to the proportions below the threshold (U.S. Bureau of the Census, 1993). Some epidemiologic studies have analyzed mortality rates in relation to income in multiples (e.g., 150% or 200%) of the poverty threshold (Chapter 4). Income relative to the poverty threshold is a criterion for eligibility for various public assistance programs (discussed in this chapter).

Poverty rates are not the only measures of income compiled by the Bureau of the Census. For some analyses presented in this book, the distribution of household incomes for blacks in specific metropolitan areas also are examined. However, poverty rates are highly correlated with other measures of income and have the advantage of taking into account household size as well as adjustments for inflation.

Using disposable income (instead of income prior to taxes) in defining poverty would increase the number of "working poor" but reduce the poverty rate for those receiving public assistance; the national poverty rate in 1992 would increase from 14.5% (by the old method) to 18.1% (Anon., 1995a). A major departure would be the proposed annual updating of the poverty thresholds on the basis of consumer spending patterns for food, clothing, and housing during the previous 3 years (Anon., 1995a).

Poverty, income, and "self-sufficiency" do not capture all of the meaning of "social class." The development of multidimensional concepts of social class or socioeconomic status was influenced by the sociologist M. Weber (1864–1920), who proposed considering the political and status dimensions of social class in addition to economic aspects measured by income, education, and occupation. These variables are intercorrelated to some extent.

Social class is correlated with a variety of other factors (Adler et al., 1994) such as individual psychological, psychosocial, and psychodynamic variables (depression, hostility, and sense of control) and individual behavior (including health behavior). Variables at the community or societal level include residential characteristics (such as quality of air, water, housing, and neighborhood), access to health care, community norms regarding behavior (including health-related behavior), work environment, and community political and economic power structures. Many of these variables are considered later with reference to "concentration" or "neighborhood" effects of segregation. It is obvious that social class and its correlates may influence health status and mortality.

Epidemiologic Perspectives on Poverty

Poverty has been described, albeit metaphorically, as a "disease" or even "the deadliest plague" (Yankauer, 1989). At the least, it is associated with various factors more directly related to the causes of many diseases, as well as access to and quality of medical care. The U.S. Public of Health Services' Year 2000 national objectives (1991) include health outcomes (such as mortality rates) and health-related behaviors for poor persons, but not reductions in poverty rates. Presumably, it was not considered appropriate for public health agencies to lobby for changes in poverty prevalence.

If poverty or low social class is closely related to health outcomes, it seems reasonable to suggest that epidemiologists and public health administrators be more concerned with the distributions and determinants of poverty itself. Poverty or low income could be treated as a risk factor or marker for disease, analogous to physical inactivity. Consideration of poverty often involves culture-laden and moralistic definitions of subgroups, such as the "undeserving" poor (as confessed by Mr. Doolittle in "My Fair Lady") or "shiftlessness" (as discussed later). With regard to physical inactivity, terms include "laziness" and the colloquial "couch potato." Studies by sociologists (Jencks and Peterson, 1991) have involved approaches resembling epidemiologic methods but without the techniques and terminology of epidemiology.

The distribution of poverty can be described (as a "disease" or risk factor for disease) according to characteristics related to person, place, and time (Mac-Mahon and Pugh, 1970). "Rates" (i.e., prevalence rates) of poverty (as defined by the Census Bureau) are often analyzed.

Person

Characteristics of persons include age, gender, and race or ethnic group. The proportion of persons living below the federal poverty level, or the "poverty rate," is a "prevalence rate" in epidemiologic terms. Poverty rates for 1990, based on income in 1989, and the proportions of all poor persons accounted for by selected subgroups of the population are shown in Table 3-1. While these data are a snapshot of a changing situation, such as declining poverty rates for the elderly and increasing rates for children and young adult males (Jencks and Peterson, 1991; Jencks, 1991, 1993), the poverty rate among blacks was 32%; blacks comprised 29% of all poor persons in 1990, and figures for 1980 were similar (Table 3-2). In fact, poverty rates for both blacks and whites in 1990 were similar to those around 1975 (Table 3-2). According to data from the U.S. Bureau of the Census (1995), the black/white ratio of poverty rates declined slightly from 1990 to 1994 (Table 3-2); from 1993 to 1994, the absolute

Table 3-1. Descriptive epidemiology of poverty in the United States, 1990

Characteristic	Number of poor persons (in thousands)	Poverty rate (percent)	Percent of all poor persons
PERSON			
Race			
All	33,585	13.5	100.0
White	22,326	10.7	66.5
Black	9,837	31.9	29.3
Hispanic origin	6,006	28.1	17.9
Age			
<15	11,802	21.4	35.1
15–24	5,594	16.1	16.7
25–44	8,469	10.4	25.2
45–54	2,002	7.8	6.0
55–59	963	9.0	1.9
60–64	1,078	10.3	3.2
65+	3,658	12.2	10.9
Family structure			
All persons in families	25,232	12.0	75.1
Female householder, no husband	12,578	37.2	37.5
PLACE			
In metropolitan areas			
Total	24,510	12.7	73.0
In central cities	14,254	19.0	42.4
Outside central cities	10,255	8.7	30.5
Outside metropolitan areas	9,075	16.3	27.0
Non-farm vs. farm			
Non-farm	33,051	13.6	98.4
Farm	534	11.2	1.6
Region			
Northeast	5,794	11.4	17.3
Midwest	7,458	12.4	22.2
South	13,456	15.8	40.1
West	6,877	13.0	20.5
State			
Highest rate (Mississippi)		25.7	—
Lowest rate (Connecticut)		6.0	—

Data are from the U.S. Bureau of the Census (1991a).

number of poor blacks declined slightly, while the number of poor whites showed no change. However, these data obscure important regional differences in black poverty rates, as discussed later.

Black–white differences in income persist within educational levels. In the 1990 Census the proportion of families below the poverty level was 23% for whites and 39% for blacks when the householder had less than 8 years of education. Larger differences were found at higher levels of education and even

Table 3-2. Poverty rates and relative income levels
of U.S. blacks and whites

	Poverty rate			Median relative income		
Year	Black	White	Black/white	Black	White	Black/white
1959	55.1	18.1	3.0	NA*	NA	NA
1966	41.8	11.3	3.7	0.52	1.06	0.49
1970	33.5	9.9	3.4	0.58	1.05	0.55
1975	31.3	9.7	3.2	0.59	1.05	0.56
1980	32.5	10.2	3.2	0.58	1.06	0.55
1985	31.3	11.4	2.7	0.58	1.06	0.55
1990	31.9	10.7	3.0	0.60	1.06	0.57
1994	30.6	11.7	2.6	NA	NA	NA

Data are from the U.S. Bureau of the Census (1991a, b, 1995).
*NA, Data not available.

among families in which the householder had 1 or more years of college (poverty rate 3% for whites vs. 12% for blacks) according to the U.S. Bureau of the Census' Current Population Survey (*Statistical Abstract of the United States: 1994*). The distribution of number of years of education differs for blacks and whites within such broad categories as "1+ yrs. of college"; the proportion of high school (but not college) graduates has increased in recent decades among black adults (Jencks, 1991).

The highest poverty rates in 1990 for categories in Table 3-1 were for female householder families (31.1%) and for the subgroup of such families with related children <5 years old (i.e., 57.4%). For single-parent families poverty rates have averaged about 50% since 1965; if welfare benefits are not included in income, rates are even higher (Bane and Ellwood, 1989). Time trends in rates of out-of-wedlock births (per 100 or 1,000 live births) by racial and ethnic groups have been complex but remain higher among blacks than whites, although the number of white out-of-wedlock births surpassed that of blacks around 1980 (Besharov, 1996). These sociocultural phenomena are poorly understood by sociologists (as discussed later).

Poverty rate is an absolute measure of income, independent of the distribution of income in the population. Another measure of income is relative income (Table 3-2), which measures an individual's distance from the median of the income distribution for the entire nation adjusted for differences in family size (U.S. Bureau of the Census, 1991b). The median relative income was 1.05 for whites versus 0.59 for blacks in 1974; it was virtually unchanged in 1989 (i.e., 1.06 for whites vs. 0.60 for blacks) (Table 3-2).

Changes in poverty rates or average (and median) income over time for blacks and whites provide limited information on the distribution of incomes. The Gini index, or index of income concentration, is derived by ranking incomes for persons or families in the population from lowest to highest and dividing the distribution into groups of equal size such as quintiles (i.e., five equal-sized groups). The aggregate total income of each group is divided by the overall total income of all groups to yield a single measure of dispersion of income. Theoretically, the index ranges from 0 (or complete equality) to 1 (or complete inequality, where one subgroup or quintile receives all the income). The Gini index has increased progressively since about 1968 for both blacks and whites, but the black–white difference increased through the early 1990s. Studies of mortality rates in various countries have used data on inequality of income distribution (Chapter 4).

Place and Place–Time Interactions

In the 1990 Census, the prevalence of poverty (based on income for 1989) was slightly greater in the South (15.7%) than in the entire United States (13.1%) and lowest in the Northeast (10.6%) (U.S. Bureau of the Census, 1991a, 1993). However, extremely high poverty rates among blacks are found in certain urban areas outside the South. According to one definition, "ghettos" are areas with an overall poverty prevalence of greater than 40%, regardless of racial and ethnic composition (Jargowsky and Bane, 1991), while Wilson (1991b) used a definition of at least a 40% poverty rate. These definitions contrast with those based on racial and ethnic composition, leading to confusion of the term "ghettoization," which also may be used to indicate rising proportions of black residents.

The definition of ghettos as areas with more than 40% poverty rate was somewhat arbitrary but was found to correspond to subjective visual assessments of "deteriorated" urban areas (Jargowsky and Bane, 1991). In *The New American Ghetto*, sociologist-photojournalist C.J. Vergara (1995) defended the use of "ghetto" despite the concern by some "teachers, social workers, and advocates of the poor" that it overemphasizes "victimization and social pathology." The word itself was found inscribed on the walls of some areas photographed by Vergara.

Most remarkably, in 1980, 21% of all poor black persons (or 1.6 million) lived in ghettos (i.e., census tracts with poverty rates >40%), in contrast with only 2% of all poor non-Hispanic whites.

Reports from the 1990 Census used the term "poverty areas" (rather than "ghetto"), which were defined as census tracts with a poverty rate of 20% or greater. In 1990, about 37.3% of poor persons lived in poverty areas, and the majority of these (59%) lived in central cities (U.S. Bureau of the Census, 1991a). Blacks living in cities, regardless of poverty status, were more highly concentrated in poverty areas than whites or persons of Hispanic origin (who may be of any "race"). About 53.5% of *all* blacks living in central cities lived in poverty areas, and 66.9% of *poor* blacks living in central cities were concentrated in poverty areas; comparable figures for whites were 16.9% and 41.0%. These proportions are much higher than those obtained by using "ghetto" tracts (i.e., those with an overall poverty rate of >40%).

While "poor" blacks living in "ghetto" census tracts comprise only a small proportion of all "poor" blacks, the declining appropriateness of the official poverty thresholds (mentioned earlier) results in considerable underestimation of the proportion of blacks living in extremely low-income areas, especially in the Northeast and Midwest (Wilson, 1991b).

While ghettos have been defined on the basis of poverty rates by census tract, MSAs (defined in Chapter 2) are used extensively in this book. As has been true historically, in 1990 the poverty rate was higher in nonmetropolitan areas (outside MSAs) than in metropolitan areas (in MSAs) (Table 3-1). However, the majority (58.2%) of poor *metropolitan* residents lived in central cities of MSAs in 1990.

Poverty rates are published for specific MSAs and PMSAs (defined in Chapter 2), as well as for smaller units including counties, census tracts, and census-block groups. While national poverty rates for blacks changed little between 1970 and 1980 (Table 3-2), black–white differences in underemployment have increased among young adults in many inner cities during this period (Lichter, 1988). A number of large MSAs in the Northeast and Midwest showed increases in poverty rates for blacks during the 1970s and 1980s (Farley, 1991; Jencks and Pederson, 1991; Wilson, 1987, 1991b). A few MSAs in the Northeast and Midwest had black poverty rates that approached (or, for Milwaukee, reached) 40% in 1990 (Table 3-3). New Orleans was the only southern MSA with such a high black poverty rate, although few southern MSAs are shown in Table 3-3 because few had total populations of more than 1 million in 1980. With a few exceptions (New Orleans and a few MSAs in Florida), MSAs with poverty rates above 30% in 1990 were in the Northeast and Midwest, where the highest segregation indexes and the smallest declines in segregation also occurred (Chapter 2). The combination of these trends perpetuates or even increases the geographic concentration of poverty rates in the inner cities of these urban areas (Massey and Denton, 1993).

The number of ghetto poor in metropolitan areas increased by 29.5% from 1970 to 1980 (from 1.89 to 2.45 million), with a larger increase among Hispanics than blacks, but the proportion of all poor persons living in ghettos increased slightly for blacks but not Hispanics (Jargowsky and Bane, 1991). Most of these overall increases were due to a limited number of urban areas (MSAs) in the Northeast and Midwest regions, while ghetto poverty declined in southern MSAs. In fact, the large increases in ghetto poverty for blacks from 1970 to 1980 for New York City, Chicago, Philadelphia, Detroit, and Newark accounted for most of the increase in ghetto poverty among all U.S. blacks during this period (Jargowsky and Bane, 1991).

The author's compilation of census data for individual tracts in 1970 and 1990 for these selected large cities shows a large increase between 1970 and 1990 in the number of blacks living in tracts where the *black* poverty rate was more than 40% in New York City (five counties) and Chicago (Chicago City and Chicago Heights combined) (Table 3-4). This measure changed little in Philadelphia, where the black poverty rate and segregation index for the entire MSA also showed little change. The most dramatic change in number of blacks living in what might be termed "black ghettos" was in Detroit (Detroit City), where both the black poverty rate and the segregation index of the MSA increased between 1970 and 1990. Large MSAs in the Northeast

Table 3-3. Trends in poverty rates for blacks, and segregation index in 1990, in 38 MSAs with >1 million total population in 1980

MSA*	Black poverty rate 1970	1980	1990	Percent change 1980–1990	1970–1990	Black–white segregation 1990
Anaheim	17	16	10	−39	−41	43
Atlanta	29	26	22	−14	−24	73
Baltimore	26	27	23	−14	−12	75
Boston	27	26	22	−15	−19	70
Buffalo	28	33	37	+13	+32	84
Chicago	24	35	30	−13	+25	87
Cincinnati	30	33	34	+4	+12	80
Cleveland	25	29	31	+8	+24	86
Columbus	25	24	29	+23	+14	71
Dallas	31	25	27	+6	−13	66
Denver	25	18	25	+34	0	66
Detroit	22	29	33	+14	+50	89
Fort Lauderdale	31	29	27	−9	−13	73
Houston	31	22	28	+25	−10	69
Indianapolis	23	29	26	−8	+13	80
Kansas City	27	25	28	+12	+4	76
Los Angeles	24	18	21	+17	−13	71
Miami	32	31	30	−1	−6	75
Milwaukee	27	35	41	+17	+58	84
Minneapolis	24	27	37	+40	+54	65
Nassau and Suffolk Counties, NY	19	17	12	−28	−37	79
New Orleans	43	38	41	+8	−5	74
New York, NY	23	29	25	−13	+9	78
Newark	23	29	20	−31	−13	83
Philadelphia	25	30	26	−16	+4	82
Phoenix	30	18	27	+49	−25	51
Pittsburgh	30	27	36	+31	+20	75
Portland, OR	27	23	29	+28	+7	68
Riverside	24	27	20	−24	−17	49
Sacramento	27	26	24	−8	−11	58
St. Louis	31	30	31	+5	0	81
San Antonio	36	29	26	−9	−28	57
San Diego	23	18	21	+18	−9	59
San Francisco	23	18	23	+28	0	65
San Jose	15	15	13	−12	−13	45
Seattle	21	21	22	+5	+5	60
Tampa	39	35	33	−6	−15	74
Washington, DC	18	17	13	−26	−28	68

Data on poverty rates are from reports of the U.S. Bureau of the Census on individual MSA. Data on segregation indexes are from Farley and Frey (1992, 1994).

*Names are abbreviated.

Table 3-4. Changes in numbers of blacks living in census tracts with >40% black poverty rate in five large urban areas*

Place and year	Total poor blacks (A)	Blacks in census tracts with >40% black poverty (B)	(B/A) × 100	Black poverty (percent)	Segregation index
NEW YORK, NY					
1970	399,021	50,690	12.7	23	73
1990	544,144	186,145	34.2	25	78
CHICAGO					
1970	276,951	74,951	27.1	24	89
1990	358,798	190,078	53.0	30	87
PHILADELPHIA					
1970	165,121	55,674	33.7	25	83
1990	179,191	62,690	35.0	26	82
NEWARK					
1970	13,343	56,344	23.7	23	75
1990	19,368	45,485	42.6	20	83
DETROIT					
1970	24,000	142,569	16.8	22	81
1990	157,303	270,812	58.1	33	89

*Segregation indexes for 1970 are from Massey and Denton (1993) and for 1990, from Farley and Frey (1994a); both are based on census block groups as the units of the MSA. Other sources are census reports for 1970 and 1990; numbers of blacks living in census tracts with black poverty rate >40% were added.

and Midwest are of particular interest in analyses of mortality rates (Chapter 5).

Some Correlates and Consequences of Poverty for Blacks

Public Assistance Programs and Poverty Paradoxes

The U.S. Bureau of the Census provides data on participation in public assistance programs according to various characteristics such as sex, age, and region of the country (U.S. Bureau of the Census, 1992a). Included in these reports are Aid for Families with Dependent Children (AFDC) and the Special Supplemental Food Program for Women, Infants, and Children (WIC). Other programs that are relevant to this book include public or subsidized rental housing (discussed with reference to public housing and segregation) and Medicaid.

"Welfare" is often used only with reference to AFDC. Blacks comprised a declining proportion of welfare recipients in the 1970s to 1980s (Peterson, 1991), although the proportion of recipients remains higher for blacks than whites. WIC includes a large proportion of the population with limited access to primary care, with about 43% of all infants (72% in New York City) enrolled (Birkhead et al., 1995). Poor populations in inner-city (and rural) areas are especially well represented, and WIC has included not only nutritional programs but efforts to immunize children against measles and other infectious diseases. There is considerable evidence that public assistance programs have a beneficial impact on health, especially with regard to AFDC and WIC, as well as Medicaid, by affecting adverse pregnancy outcomes (Chapter 6).

Head Start was initiated for preschool children in 1965 as part of the War on Poverty. It is mentioned because two-thirds of children served are minorities, and many participating families are headed by single parents who also receive AFDC (and Medicaid). Despite evidence for positive effects (including gains in nutrition, motor development, and immunization coverage), the majority of eligible children in the United States are not included in Head Start, which was budgeted at $2.8 billion in fiscal year 1993 (Zigler et al., 1994; Zigler and Styfco, 1996).

The apparent failure of federal programs to reduce the national poverty rate is called the "poverty paradox" (Peterson, 1991). However, while public assistance payments increased during the 1970s, costs of antipoverty programs are small compared with other federal budget items (Jencks, 1993). Social Security and Medicare, which are not "means tested," are very costly but are not targeted to the poor. The same considerations also hold for the persistence of the black–white gap in poverty rates. While blacks participate disproportionately in means-tested programs, the benefits are rarly high enough to lift beneficiaries (even those in multiple public assistance programs) out of poverty. Also, national surveys show that persons in such programs still suffer from inadequacies in clothing and housing, though perhaps less often with regard to food. Within two broad income levels (<20,000 and >20,000) blacks experienced such problems more often than whites (Blendon et al., 1995).

Economic recessions have dampened any impact of public assistance programs on poverty rates, and the greater susceptibility of blacks since the 1930s is well known (Massey and Denton, 1993). During the 1990–1991 recession, blacks were less likely than whites to "exit" from poverty, and nonpoor blacks were more likely to become poor than nonpoor whites (i.e., 6.5% vs. 2.5%) (Bureau of the Census, 1993). The poorly understood increase in households headed by women, especially among blacks (noted earlier), has also blunted the impact of any increases in spending on antipoverty programs. However, tangential to the poverty issue, the black middle class, long ago described by W.E.B. Du Bois (Lewis, 1993), did expand, especially in the 1960s and 1970s, and inequalities in income distributions among blacks have increased.

Health Insurance

In Bureau of the Census publications, health insurance is specified as private (commercial) health insurance, Medicaid, Medicare, and various veterans programs. With the exception of Medicare (a "universal" program), social class differences explain black–white differences in health insurance coverage, especially prior to age 65 years. Health insurance coverage is very strongly associated with income level. The Bureau of the Census reported that, in 1994, 11.1 million (or 29%) of all poor persons had no health insurance; this rate was about twice that for all persons, and poor persons comprised 28% of all the uninsured (vs. about 14% of the total population in 1990; Table 3-1). Among *poor* persons in the 1990 Census, the proportions not covered by health insurance were 30.6% for whites, 24.3% for blacks, and 41.3% for Hispanics; in contrast, among *all* persons, the figures for the same three racial and ethnic groups were 12.9%, 19.7%, and 32.4% (U.S. Bureau of the Census, 1991a). For Hispanics, type of occupation (or probability of employer coverage of health insurance) and immigration status affect health insurance status (Valdez et al., 1993).

Because participation in Medicare is not means tested, it is referred to as "social insurance" while Medicaid is often regarded as "welfare" (Tilson et al., 1995). Despite universal eligibility, a reverse means test for Part B of Medicare is the ability to pay the monthly premiums for subsidized supplemental medical care involving physician services (not covered by Part A, which relates to hospital services). The impact of Medicare (introduced in 1965) on health is uncertain because analyses of time trends in health indicators are difficult to interpret (Kuller, 1988). In Los Angeles, however, Medicare resulted in a decline in the proportion of elderly patients seen at public hospitals, which tend to serve the poor and uninsured in that city, presumably due to a shift toward use of private hospitals (Glassman et al., 1994). This finding suggests that national or state plans for health insurance coverage of currently uninsured persons (of all age groups) may have consequences for the resource needs of public hospitals, often located in poor, inner city areas with large minority populations.

The introduction of Medicaid (in 1966) resulted in increased use of health services, probably with a beneficial impact on the health of the population, including poor children (Orr et al., 1988). Also, Medicaid expansion (in 1987) to near-universal coverage for low-income pregnant women and infants (i.e., pregnant women with family incomes 133% of the federal poverty level, or higher in some states) has provided an opportunity to assess the potential impact of universal health insurance on the burden of uncompensated care by hospitals (Dubay et al., 1995).

Lack of health insurance is associated with poorer self-perceived health status (Franks et al., 1993) and with high hospitalization rates for chronic conditions, reflecting poor access to primary care that might have prevented the need for hospitalization (Bindman et al., 1995) and reduced the chance of dying from "preventable" diseases (Chapter 4). Differential treatment of black and white Medicaid and Medicare patients, even after adjustment for social class differences, are discussed later (Chapter 6). Finally, studying the impact of the expansion of managed care programs to Medicaid and AFDC recipients (in many states) on health outcomes is of great interest (Chapter 7).

Homelessness

In a review of a publication on the history of tuberculosis, homelessness was listed as one of five "interconnected epidemics," including HIV-AIDS and tuberculosis, that affected New York City and certain other urban areas after about 1979 (Dooley, 1995). Homelessness is closely associated with poverty as a potential outcome or sequela. It was mentioned with reference to critiques of large, predominantly minority, public housing projects that such projects (while involving extreme segregation and poor overall quality of life) may offer an alternative to homelessness (Chapter 2).

Results of a cross-sectional survey of homeless persons in northern California were compared with findings from other surveys of nonhomeless populations (Winkleby et al., 1992b). Even when compared with an *impoverished* domiciled group, blacks were more common among the homeless. In a study of families (defined as women with children) in New York City, those who requested shelter and who had been on welfare within the past 6 months but had not been in a shelter in the past 30 days were compared with a random sample of housed families from public assistance rolls. Despite oversampling of blacks in the control group, black were more common among those who requested shelter (Weitzman et al., 1992).

Duration of homelessness is an important consideration with regard to its potential effects on health. In a national telephone survey of a random sample of 1,507 adults, more homeless minorities were found to have been homeless for more than 1 year (Link et al., 1994). Consideration of duration of homelessness rather than prevalence at a given point in time emphasizes the magnitude of the problem. Studies have shown a higher prevalence of homelessness, at a given point in time or during a defined time period, for blacks than whites even after adjusting for income or poverty status (Susser et al., 1994). The explanations for this finding are not clear, but could involve place of residence and factors related to lack of social support from relatives or friends. The problem of hypertension control in the homeless, with their more urgent daily concerns of survival, illustrates the limits of a strict biomedical paradigm of hypertension control that ignores social problems (Kinchen and Wright, 1991). Hypertension control is a special problem for inner-city minorities.

Sociological Perspectives on Black Poverty and the Urban Underclass

While removal of all inequities by race would have limited impact on the overall problem of poverty in the United States, debates in the sociological and lay literature (as well as in the media) on the causes of poverty and the urban "underclass" appear to be strongly influenced by racial considerations. Therefore, the social and policy impact of race issues is greater than that anticipated from the proportion of poor or low-income persons that are black.

According to the *structural* view, understanding the relationship between poverty and race may require understanding how discrimination or (more broadly) racism in the "political economy" affect the "economic, social and political institutions" that have restricted the economic mobility of blacks and Hispanics (Stafford and Ladner, 1990). Despite improvement in attitudes about equal job opportunities for blacks, there has been much less support for and little change in attitudes about federal government implementation of policies for nondiscrimination in hiring (Schuman et al., 1985). The denial of an opportunity to pursue the advertised job occurred for young black men in 17% of audits in Chicago and 23% in Washington, DC (Fix and Struyk, 1993).

Also, blacks have no significant base of capital that "flows" in segregated areas (Gans, 1990). A "dual labor market" economic concept has been used by sociologists with regard to black–white differences in employment patterns. Privileged workers in the "primary" labor market (PLM) are offered opportunities for on-job training; level of education and social position influence entry into the PLM. Blacks (especially ghetto residents) are largely limited to the "secondary" labor market of domestic and fast-food services. Wilson (1987, 1991a,b) has emphasized lack of opportunities for employment due to the loss of manufacturing jobs in inner cities. The issue of the viability of businesses in inner cities as a "neighborhood" effect is discussed later.

In contrast to structural views, the anthropologist O. Lewis (1966) coined the phrase "*culture of poverty*" based on studies of poverty and family life in Mexico, San Juan (Puerto Rico), and Puerto Ricans living in New York City. Learned or "cultural" habits are transmitted from one generation to another. Although the term has been both "used and misused" in the literature, this "subculture" or "counterculture" (in sociological terms) within the predominant culture was viewed as both an adaptation and a reaction of lower-class or socially marginalized groups in certain (but not all) capitalistic societies. The subculture was characterized by feelings of fatalism, helplessness, dependence, inferiority, and widespread belief in male superiority. Lewis (1966) cited the idea that female-headed households among blacks were a legacy of slavery, but this has been shown to have no historical basis.

The idea of a static culture of poverty has received little support from two "experiments." In a "natural experiment" of near-universal employment during a period of economic growth in Boston, previously unemployed minority persons sought and obtained employment, although black–white differences in income persisted (Osterman, 1991). Employment itself is not a panacea for poverty, as witnessed by the "working poor" (Schwarz and Volgy, 1992). The second experiment, the Gatreaux project in Chicago, involved helping low-income black families to move from inner-city public housing projects to private-market housing in surrounding areas through vouchers that subsidize the higher rents. In random samples of female heads of households (mostly covered by AFDC), those who moved to the suburbs were more likely to have jobs when surveyed than those who moved within the inner city (63.8% vs. 50.9%). In multivariate models, the addition of two culture of poverty variables (low internal sense of control and long-term AFDC dependency) reduced the likelihood of employment, but being a second-generation AFDC recipient had no effect (Rosenbaum and Popkin, 1991). Other studies among blacks also have not supported an intergenerational effect of welfare dependency (Stafford and Ladner, 1990), while evidence for whites is equivocal (Duncan et al., 1988).

However, the Gatreaux project found that "fatalistic attitudes" (part of the culture of poverty syndrome) had an effect on work. The lack of opportunity for employment in the inner city was an apparent barrier to those who wanted to work, thus supporting Wilson's "spatial mismatch" idea (1987, 1991a,b). However, qualitative studies indicated that lack of public transportation and lack of social support for child care (and financial costs of replacing such care) were problems for the women who moved to the suburbs.

In another survey in Chicago (in 1987), only a very small proportion of parents 18–44 years old residing in poverty areas (20% poverty rate or higher) who were unemployed could be classified as truly "shiftless" or unwilling to work, and only a small proportion of those who did not want to work supported themselves by illegal activities. Also, among unemployed men, blacks were more willing than whites to accept low-paying jobs (Tienda and Stier, 1991). This situation may have changed in recent years, however, so that further study is needed.

The idea of a subculture of poverty has a counterpart with regard to crime and homicide in the proposed black "subculture of violence." Confounding between poverty and race in examining crime rates is often not adequately emphasized. The structurally disadvantaged position of blacks may be a more basic cause of black violence in a causal chain similar to that for whites. In urban areas, poverty rate is the most important factor associated with homicide rates, specifically for homicides involving strangers, while "percent black" (the proportion of the total population that is black) is of much less importance (Parker, 1989).

The culture of poverty idea is sometimes closely associated with the "underclass" concept (Gans, 1990). The original concept of an "under-class" (Myrdal, 1963) in rural and large urban areas, where blacks were disproportionately represented, emphasized economic conditions and not deviant behavior. If deviance is to be included as a key feature of the underclass, then the criteria must be clearly defined, but it would seem preferable to study deviance as a separate phenomenon (Gans, 1990). If extreme and persistent poverty is the only feature of the underclass, then "lower class" or "extreme lower class" could be used and clearly defined in terms of percentage of the appropriate poverty threshold (Gans, 1990, 1993; Steinberg, 1989).

Proponents of culture of poverty and of deviant underclass concepts, especially those that focus on blacks or the ghetto underclass, fail to recognize the effects of segregation on the quality of neighborhoods and "normative" behavior (Massey and Denton, 1993). However, Fuch's "ghetto ethno-underclass" (1990) underscored the legacy of segregation and social isolation for blacks, and Wilson's "ghetto underclass" (1987, 1991a,b) emphasized the lack of jobs, education, and training and the lure of the "underground economy" in the ghettos. A comprehensive approach to the urban "underclass" (including inner-city blacks) should include not only "personal responsibility" but also the need for "job training, job creation, the removal of racial stereotypes and discrimination" and the "spatial concentration of poverty" that challenge policymakers (Johnson, 1996). Even the conservative political scientist Kelso (1994), who has emphasized the "culture of poverty" and the degeneration of "values" of "underclass" blacks, supports the Gatreaux project's efforts (discussed earlier) to relocate poor inner-city blacks from segregated areas to the suburbs in Chicago.

"Concentration" or "Neighborhood" Effects

Civil Disturbances in Ghettos:
Symptoms of "Concentration" or "Neighborhood" Effects

In the United States, urban civil disturbances that followed the assassination of Martin Luther King Jr. contributed to the passage of the 1968 Fair Housing Act as an amendment to a bill dealing with the prosecution of participants in the riots. The Kerner Commission report (Kerner, 1968) recognized segregation as an underlying factor in the riots. The optimism that followed the 1968 Fair Housing Act was short lived as difficulties in its enforcement became evident. The 1988 amendments, which provided more power to HUD and the Attorney General, have been restricted and their future is uncertain (Massey and Denton, 1993).

The comprehensive evaluation of the social, economic, political, educational, and health status of U.S. blacks by Jaynes and Williams (1989), *A Common Destiny: Blacks and American Society*, included a prediction that the "surface calm" in some urban areas in the 1980s could rapidly vanish. The litany of "ingredients" for civil disturbance identified in 1989 (uncanny, in view of the Los Angeles riots of 1992), included "large populations of jobless youths, an extensive sense of relative deprivation and injustice, distrust of the legal system, frequently abrasive police–community relations, highly visible inequalities, extreme concentrations of poverty, and great racial awareness." Highlighted as a basis for "social turbulence" was the "widespread dissatisfaction with the operation of the criminal justice system," which was perceived as being "too lenient with whites who commit offenses against blacks" (Jaynes and Williams, 1989, p. 30).

After the riots of 1992 in Los Angeles, related initially to perceived police injustice, a commission reached the same conclusions as previous commissions created after previous riots. The 1968 report on civil disorders, with O. Kerner as Chairman and J.V. Lindsay as Vice Chairman, identified the underlying conditions contributing to riots (Kerner, 1968). The Kerner Commission report quoted President Johnson's national address in June 1967, which indicated that the "conditions that breed despair and violence" were well known, including "discrimination, slums, poverty, disease, [and] not enough jobs." K.B. Clark's comments in the Kerner Commission report, still appropriate today, were that the commissions on riots in 1919 in Chicago, in Harlem in 1935 and 1943, and in Watts in 1965 produced "the same analyses, the same recommendations, and the same inaction."

The involvement of Latinos, representing about half of those arrested, in the 1992 Los Angeles riots has been interpreted as a response to breakdown in municipal order rather than the result of participation with blacks in social protest (Hayes-Bautista et al., 1993). In 1992, the reactions of many whites (especially politicians) emphasized the lawlessness and property damage, but rarely mentioned the underlying problems of the ghetto. M.L. King Jr.'s fear of "cycles of chaos and destruction" is still salient, because the causes of the underlying black "rage" have not been addressed (West, 1994).

A secondary effect of the 1992 Los Angeles riots was reduced access to health care due to closure of health clinics, physicians' offices, and supportive institutions (Fong, 1995). More important than civil disturbances, from a public health perspective, are the chronic problems in ghettos such as exposure to high levels of noise and stress, crime and violence, poor housing, inadequate services (e.g., food, recreation, and medical care), harmful substances in the occupational and general ambient environment, crowing, infectious agents, and illicit drug use.

"Neighborhood" Effects and Ghetto Counterculture

The development of black urban "underclass" communities in America has been detailed by Massey and Denton (1993), who emphasized the role of black–white residential segregation in the creation of a counterculture called the "culture of segregation." In the "spiral" of decline due to the concentration of blacks in high-poverty areas, social problems proliferate, such as crime, drugs, physical deterioration of buildings and environment, poor access to goods and services (as well as jobs), and more complex changes in behavioral norms and attitudes. Examples of the counterculture include the "norm" of single-parent families on welfare and a "baby club culture" (Massey and Denton, 1993). Only a few "neighborhood" or "concentration" effects of segregation are discussed here.

Mention is made of illicit drug use by blacks because it is affected by both ethnicity and neighborhood characteristics. A study of trends in cocaine use by pregnant women shows diversity within the "black" population (Chapter 2), with lower use among foreign-born than American-born blacks at an inner-city hospital in New York City in 1988–1992 (McCalla et al., 1995). More important, an analysis of data from the 1988 U.S. National Household Survey of Drug Abuse suggested that apparent racial and ethnic differences in crack cocaine use may reflect neighborhood factors. Respondents were stratified into local areas defined by aggregates of city blocks to control for "neighborhood factors." After such control the estimated relative odds of crack use was not higher for African Americans or Hispanics than for whites (Lillie-Blanton et al., 1995). The findings were generalizable only to persons living in racially mixed neighborhoods with at least one crack smoker and could differ from those with "total racial segregation." However, it is clear that perceptions of social problems based on race can be very misleading if social class and neighborhood effects are not considered.

Ideas for studies of urban African Americans have been suggested by the results of national household surveys of drug abuse among Hispanics. Among Mexican-American Hispanic participants in surveys conducted in 1988–1991, crack cocaine smoking was reported less frequently by those choosing to be interviewed in Spanish rather than English even after "neighborhood" effects were controlled by stratifying the respondents. This suggested that strong identification with culture of origin among Mexican Americans may be protective against illicit drug use (Wagner-Echeagaray et al., 1994). Similar studies are needed among inner-city black youths using "acculturation" or ethnic identification scales (Chapter 2). Neighborhood characteristics could interact with other factors such as degree of ethnic identification or identification with "Afrocentrism" versus counterculture values.

The apparent paucity of "black entrepreneurs" in inner cities or "urban underclass" areas relative to certain other racial and ethnic groups (Kelso, 1994) may be due largely to a "concentration" effect overlooked by many conservative adherents to culture of poverty theories. While some growth of "minority" business establishments has occurred in Los Angeles, major obstacles remain, especially for blacks desiring entrepreneurship in central city areas. Recent Supreme Court decisions regarding government contracts with minority business are involved, but "institutional" barriers (discrimination) include inadequate support from financial institutions due in part to their reluctance to provide insurance coverage for business enterprises in poor central city areas plagued by social problems (Johnson, 1996).

General redevelopment in downtown Los Angeles has done little to improve the quality of life in the South-Central area, damaged during the 1992 civil unrest. Jobless rates for black males reach 50%, and "low-level service and custodial jobs" are usually filled by newly arriving Latino immigrants (Johnson, 1996). Also, a lack of attractiveness of such jobs may occur in the ghetto "culture of segregation" (Massey and Denton, 1993). Perceptions and attitudes about black culture in ghettos by some whites probably adversely impact on employment chances for blacks (Hacker, 1995; Jencks, 1993; Wilson, 1991a,b). The roles of prejudice and stereotyping, however, need more study.

A temporal movement of ghetto cultures further away from the "mainstream" has been suggested, although depictions are influenced by such factors as sampling schemes for interviews, the theoretical perspectives of the sociologists involved, and the interpretations of others. Sociologists have observed that "old heads," or those who work for low wages (e.g., at fast-food restaurants), are becoming more rare (Massey and Denton, 1993). Such persons do not fit the "cool" image (imprecisely defined) by the "street culture" of the ghetto (Connor, 1995). In *Slim's Table* (1992), sociologist M. Duneier concluded that, in contrast to the "old ghetto," the "norm" in Chicago South Side ghettos had become a counterculture, with violence and a decline in "social order." Blacks who did not conform to this new norm were becoming more isolated.

On the other hand, the "values" and "culture" of black youths surviving in inner cities may be overgeneralized (Henry, 1990; hooks, 1995) and may be viewed as (in part) exaggerations of the values of the larger society (Duneier, 1992; Kelso, 1994). For example, broad sociocultural trends in attitudes in the United States, as well as a decline in the pool of marriageable black men and relatively lesser economic gains from marriage for black than white women, probably contribute to the ghetto "norm" of unwed motherhood (Tucker and Mitchell-Kernan, 1995). In a television interview, a lottery-ticket buyer crystallized the "American dream" as the quest "to get the big bucks easy." How do such societal attitudes contribute to the lure of selling illicit drugs in high-unemployment areas of inner cities? Also, society permits federal subsidizing of addictive and harmful tobacco products, considered as "gateway" agents in the genesis of drug addiction, as well as corporate tax deductions for an advertising and marketing assault that often targets minorities in inner cities (Chapter 6).

The importance of high-school dropout rates (Chapter 1) in the development of underclass behavior in ghettos has been emphasized in programs (mostly private, nongovernment-sponsored) aimed at "nurturing" young black males. These programs focus on adolescent development or "socialization" and the role of Afrocentrism (Mincy, 1993). Black male youths in inner cities may have become "demonized in the popular mind" to an extent not previously experienced by any other group, especially after the 1992 Los Angeles riots (Loury, 1996). However, ethnographers studying cocaine use in inner cities have been interested not only in "deviants" but also in those who survive in deleterious environments (Holden, 1989). The potential for a greater role of black churches has been advocated (Jencks, 1992; Loury, 1996).

Conclusion

Persistently higher overall poverty rates for blacks than whites, along with both black–white segregation and social class segregation, result in the concentration of urban blacks in "ghettos" or "poverty areas." The "ghetto" threshold of 40% poverty rate is subjective, and more descriptive work appears to be needed on quality of life for blacks (and whites) in neighborhoods (census tracts or block groups) with somewhat lower poverty rates (for example, 20%–40%). Ghetto poverty is only a part of the total problem of black poverty. but it influences debates about poverty, welfare, homelessness, universal health insurance, and the underclass.

Highly segregated (or "hypersegregated") urban areas with dwindling economic opportunities perpetuate "concentration effects" on work and life opportunities for blacks and a "ghetto underclass" (Wilson, 1991a,b) or a "culture of segregation" (Massey and Denton, 1993). These conditions are related to the macrosocial constraints of isolation in poor ghetto areas, especially in the Northeast and Midwest regions. They may also be relevant to the health of blacks.

The next chapter examines poverty in relation to mortality rates for blacks and black–white differences in mortality rates, and it introduces the epidemiology of American apartheid by comparison of mortality rates in South Africa and America and by examination of variations in death rates among U.S. metropolitan areas that could be related to the level of segregation (Chapter 4).

4

From Socioeconomic Epidemiology toward the Epidemiology of American Apartheid

The conceptual framework in Chapter 1 involves consideration of the effects of social class on the health of blacks and the possibility of a combined effect of black poverty and the segregation of blacks in urban areas ("concentration" or "neighborhood" effects). In this chapter, the results of a few studies of the relationship between poverty (or, more broadly, social class) and mortality are outlined, including the pioneering work of Kitagawa and Hauser (1973) on "socioeconomic epidemiology." The extension of this field to encompass segregation as a variable in predicting variation in mortality rates for blacks, and black/white ratios of mortality rates, is introduced, to be followed by detailed analyses in Chapter 5.

Socioeconomic Epidemiology

General Studies

The relationship between social class and risk of illness and death has a long history, including the observations of R. Virchow (1821–1902) on epidemics in Upper Silesia, with his belief in the relevance of "liberty, education and prosperity" to health (Silver, 1987; Susser, 1983, 1985). This topic is receiving increasing attention in epidemiology, sociology, and psychology (e.g., Adler et al., 1994; Liberatos et al., 1988; Marmot et al., 1987; Susser, 1985). Statistical studies started in Europe, due to the availability of data on occupational or other social-class indicators as well as better systems of registration of the population, and this tradition has continued (Susser, 1983, 1985; Marmot et al., 1991; Vagero, 1991).

In Britain evidence indicates a widening gap in health and mortality between **53** the "occupational classes" starting in the early 1950s, as documented in the Black Research Working Group report of 1980 and by Townsend (1990). A somewhat similar trend occurred in the United States (discussed later). The degree of inequality in the distribution of income (Chapter 3) has been used in other studies of mortality. In contrast to Britain, Japan has had a narrowing of income distribution since about 1970 and an increase in absolute life expectancy and in life expectancy relative to Britain and to other countries (Wilkinson 1992).

Social class, like race and ethnicity, is a multidimensional variable (Chapter 3), and social class indicators can change over time. While occupational groupings have the advantage of being used consistently over many decades, a single factor cannot capture the meaning of social class (Krieger and Fee, 1994). Often education alone is used because it may be the only variable available and also may be relatively comparable in meaning across countries. Also, education is sometimes more strongly related to health outcomes than other social class indicators. A review of studies on mortality differences by education among men 35–64 years old in nine westernized countries showed that inequalities in mortality rates were smaller in the Netherlands, Sweden, Denmark, and Norway than in the United States, France, and Italy. Finland, England, and Wales were intermediate. The strength of the association between education and mortality was similar across countries, but the size of the educational inequalities varied (Kunst and Mackenbach, 1994). As noted earlier (Chapter 3), inequalities in the income distribution are also smaller in Scandinavian countries than in the United States.

In the United States, the term "socioeconomic epidemiology" was introduced by Kitagawa and Hauser (1973), who used data on educational level, income, and occupation to show the association between social class or socioeconomic status and age-adjusted mortality (from all causes of death combined). It had not previously been possible to compute death rates by education or income level directly from official U.S. tabulations of deaths, because social class variables were not reported on the death record. Kitagawa and Hauser's work (1973) was based on the "1960 Matched Records Study," which was a special effort that involved linkage of 1960 Census records on the income and educational level of individuals with death certificates (from the National Center for Health Statistics) for persons 25 years of age or older in 1960. Some 340,000 deaths in 1960 were linked with the 1960 Census records.

Kitagawa and Hauser (1973) found a stronger association between mortality and education than income when both variables were considered together. Using the data published by Kitagawa and Hauser (1973), along with more recent data from a national sample, Pappas et al. (1993) showed an even stronger association in 1986 than in 1960 for both whites and blacks.

Poor health immediately prior to death may result in a decline in income, thereby affecting studies of the association between mortality and income-based social class variables. Kitagawa and Hauser (1973) discussed the "reverse causal path," or the effect of health on income, in some detail. They compared the strength of the association between income and mortality within specific age categories, because any effect of health status on income would be greatest for persons of "working age." Kitagawa and Hauser (1973) also compared the associations with mortality based on income with those based on education, because the latter would be less affected by "drift." Their results provided some limited support (for some age groups) for the "reverse causal path," resulting in overestimation of the association between income and mortality, but subsequent research has provided no evidence for a strong effect (Adler et al., 1994).

The association between low maternal education and higher risk of infant mortality reported by Antonovsky and Bernstein (1977) has been confirmed. Birth records that include information on maternal and paternal education must be linked with death records in order to estimate infant mortality rates by maternal education for individual births. In an analysis of several linked data sets, from 1964–1966 and 1987, infant mortality rate was strongly (inversely) associated with maternal education in both blacks and whites (Singh and Yu, 1995). Although infant mortality rates declined from 1964–1966 to 1987, the gradient in these rates by maternal education persisted in 1987 and was larger than that in 1964–1966. This trend is consistent with findings on trends for young adults, as already mentioned. Updating some of Antonovsky and Bernstein's analyses (1977), Najman (1993) found that for eight countries (i.e., the United States, Canada, Australia, and parts of Europe) the degree of inequality in the distribution of income in a population was an important variable in infant mortality rates.

Trends in educational differentials in mortality in the United States (Feldman et al., 1989) since 1960 indicate that death rates among men declined more steadily for more educated than less educated, while for women the strong inverse association between education and mortality in 1960 remained at about the same level by the 1980s. Although mortality rates from coronary heart disease, the leading cause of death in America for many decades, were once higher in the higher social classes, the direction of the association changed to an inverse one.

Both knowledge of risk factors for coronary heart disease (overweight, hypertension, and high blood cholesterol) and actual levels of these factors in individuals were highly significantly associated with level of education, independent of income or occupation, in the Stanford Five-City Project (Winkleby et al., 1990, 1992a). This is a study of the impact of community-based health education on health outcomes in selected California cities. The results may reflect differences in lifestyle by education, but also the effects of health education and promotion programs that are more effective in reaching and influencing the more highly educated segments of a society (Najman, 1993). The latter phenomenon has been called "reverse targeting" of educational and other interventions, because the very groups in most need of interventions (low social class and minorities) are seldom reached.

One major national study has involved follow-up of participants in the the First National Health and Nutrition Examination Survey (NHANES). In the First National Epidemiologic Follow-up Study (NHEFS), some 14,407 participants 35–74 years old were examined medically in 1971–1975 (as part of

NHANES), and the cohort was followed for an average of about 10 years (Williams and Lepkowski, 1992). For men, those at or below the poverty level and near the poverty level had more than twice the death rate of those 151%–200% or more than 200% of the poverty level (see Chapter 3). After adjusting for all the risk factors measured (such as health behaviors, blood pressure, serum cholesterol, and diabetes), men at or near the poverty level still had mortality rates 1.4–1.7 times those of men with incomes 150%–200% of the poverty level. Results for women were much less striking, with the largest effect apparent (as for men) among 25–44 year olds. The addition of health-care-related variables (having health insurance and medical check-ups and using a private physician for care) to the models resulted in the removal of almost all of the effect of poverty status on health, suggesting that poverty operates through many pathways to influence mortality.

In Oakland (Alameda County), CA, health behavior factors alone could not account for the association between social class and mortality in a cohort of adults 35 years of age and older followed from 1965 to 1984 (Haan et al., 1987). A complex mixture of sociopolitical environmental factors was suggested to explain the higher mortality rates in federally designated poverty areas, including "higher crime rates, poorer housing, lack of transportation, and higher levels of environmental contaminants" (Haan et al., 1987). A similar constellation of factors may be involved in black–white differences in mortality.

Mortality Studies of U.S. Blacks and Whites

In Kitagawa and Hauser's classic study (1973), small numbers of nonwhite deaths in the study sample permitted comparison of mortality ratios for nonwhite males and females for only three categories of education, and the differences in mortality by education were not as large as for whites. For nonwhite males 25–64 years old, the mortality ratio (standardized for age) was 1.14 for 0–4 years of education and 0.87 for 9+ years. For white males 25–64 years old, the mortality ratio was 1.60 for 0–4 years of education or more than twice the ratio of 0.78 for 4 years of college (or more). These ratios are relative to the total mortality for all persons in the entire group (e.g., all white males), which was assigned a value of 1.00.

The magnitude of the black–white mortality differences was not uniform by age group. The largest disparity in death rates was for the working years of life, and the black/white ratio declined beyond middle age, reaching less than 1.00 at the oldest ages (Kitagawa and Hauser, 1973; Sutton, 1971). This reversal or "crossover" for total death rates and for major causes of death (Table 4-1) has been a consistent finding in subsequent studies. Kitagawa and Hauser (1973) focused on errors in the data as an explanation for the crossover. Frequent discrepancies have been found between ages recorded for blacks on death certificates and ages in the 1990 Census, as also found by Kitagawa and Hauser (1973) in the 1960 Census. These errors could account for at least part of the apparent crossover in death rates for blacks and whites at older ages (Holden, 1994). However, a longitudinal (cohort) study of 2,219 blacks and 1,838 whites

Table 4-1. Black/white ratios of death rates in adults by sex and age, United States, 1991

Age (years)	All causes		Heart disease		Cerebrovascular disease		Cancers	
	Male	Female	Male	Female	Male	Female	Male	Female
15–24	2.2	1.6	2.6	2.4	0.8	2.6	0.9	1.3
25–34	2.4	2.6	2.8	3.3	3.0	3.3	1.3	1.3
35–44	2.6	2.6	2.4	3.8	4.3	3.6	1.7	1.5
45–54	2.3	2.1	2.0	3.1	4.4	3.2	2.0	1.4
55–64	1.8	1.7	1.6	2.2	3.1	2.8	1.6	1.2
65–74	1.4	1.5	1.3	1.8	2.1	2.0	1.5	1.2
75–84	1.2	1.2	1.1	1.2	1.4	1.3	1.3	1.1
85+	0.9	0.9	0.8	0.9	0.9	0.9	1.2	1.1

From the National Center for Health Statistics (1994).

in the Piedmont region of North Carolina showed the familiar crossover after age 75 years, and this finding could not be "easily dismissed as attributable to inaccuracies in the data" (Guralnick et al., 1993). Another theory involves the hardiness of black survivors at older ages, referred to as "survival of the fittest" by Sutton (1971); psychosocial characteristics of black survivors (such as social support and coping responses) may be crucial.

Other methodologic issues raised in the early studies in socioeconomic epidemiology are still receiving attention, including problems with the definition of race with regard to reliability (repeatability of self-designations) and validity (i.e., biological and sociocultural meaning) (Chapter 2). Other "errors of measurement" in epidemiology (MacMahon and Pugh, 1970) include those involved in census counting of young adult blacks and other minorities, as recognized in these early studies. Considerable controversy arose over the the 1990 Census' "undercount" of poor and minority persons living in central cities due to lower rates of cooperation with governmental agencies. Estimated undercount rates indicated that black males 40–44 years old were most often missed in 1990 (perhaps by more than 15%), with rates of near 0% for ages 10–19 years and intermediate rates for ages 20–39 years (Freedman, 1991). Analyses of death rates for black men in this book include age-specific rates for young adults (15–24 through 35–44 years), as well as death rates for black women (for whom the estimated undercount was low in the 1990 Census).

A number of studies have been conducted on black–white differences in mortality after adjustment for social class. Problems due to small study populations and small numbers of deaths among blacks are common among cohort or longitudinal ("follow-up") epidemiologic studies of mortality in specific geographic areas.

Within a large city, as well as among large cities, variation in environmental conditions, in addition to large variation in black–white disparities in social class, may exist and may emerge as important in predicting the black death rate and the black/white ratio of death rates. Baltimore was mentioned in Chapter 1 with regard to neighborhood effects due to the concentration of blacks in high-poverty urban areas. In Baltimore, mortality rates were examined in census tracts (each with about 4,000 persons) by racial composition (percent black). Socioeconomic status was defined by percentage of families with incomes below the poverty level, percentage of persons 16 + years old who were unemployed, percentage of households receiving public assistance, and 1985 median household income (Henderson and Lerner, 1992). When socioeconomic status was taken into account in multiple regression models, "percent black" was still a predictor of mortality from hypertensive heart disease, cerebrovascular diseases, nephritis and related kidney diseases, and prostate cancer. This suggests an effect of race independent of social class.

Collecting detailed data on social class for several thousand individuals in a cohort study or in special samples of linked data bases is a formidable task. Assembling such data for the entire country has been an unattainable goal. Sutton (1971) and Kitagawa and Hauser (1973) noted the dearth of national data on black–white mortality and morbidity differentials "in the context of social and economic inequalities" (Sutton, 1971). The same deficiency was emphasized by Navarro in 1990 and in subsequent editorials and reviews (Anon, 1991). The 1992 edition of *Health United States* (National Center for Health Statistics, 1993) was the first to include mortality rates by education level, an indicator of social class. While a strong association was noted between total death rate and education level, "all races" were compared with "whites." The "all races" category included "Asians," while "Hispanics" can be of any race, and many Hispanics report their race as "other" in censuses (Chapter 2); these racial and ethnic groups have markedly different mortality rates. No data on blacks or on black/white ratios of death rates within education level were provided in the 1992 and 1993 reports (National Center for Health Statistics, 1993, 1994). The number of states included in the analyses of mortality by education level is increasing, and future reports may include race-specific data.

More important than these national efforts are follow-up studies of large samples of the U.S. population. The National Longitudinal Mortality Study involves black and white adults sampled from the annual Current Population Surveys conducted by the Bureau of the Census on the noninstitutionalized population; these samples involve small numbers of households relative to the total number of households in the country (as in the decennial censuses). Data on social class variables for each individual are obtained by personal or telephone interview, and deaths are ascertained through the National Center for Health Statistics' computerized National Death Index. One report from this study, involving 32,508 deaths (in 1979–1985) among a total of 500,000 whites and 50,000 blacks showed that the more than twofold difference in mortality among 25–44 year olds was reduced after adjusting for family income (in six categories). However, significant black–white differences in death rates persisted after such adjustment (Sorlie et al., 1992). The largest residual black–white differences were among men and women 25–44 years old. An update of this study included 530,507 men and women 25 years of age or older and 54,304 deaths from 1979 through 1989 (Sorlie et al., 1995). Again, the age-adjusted black/white mortality ratios were highest for ages 25–44 years (2.07) and 45–54 years (1.68). After adjustment for employment status, income, education, marital status, and household size, the ratios were reduced but still statistically significant (i.e., 1.36 and 1.28 for the two age groups, respectively).

An analysis of data from the 1986 National Mortality Follow-back Study of 18,733 persons aged 25 years and older who died in 1986 used denominators estimated from the National Health Interview Survey of 30,725 persons 25–64 years old in 1986. Black/white ratios in age-adjusted death rates (ages 25–64) within five levels of income (Pappas et al., 1993) were much lower than those reported by Sorlie et al. (1992). This apparent disagreement may be due to several factors. First, Pappas et al. (1993) presented age-adjusted death rates for ages 25–64, while Sorlie et al. showed that black/white ratios for all causes of death were much higher at younger ages (25–44 years) than for ages 45–64. This has been a consistent finding in mortality studies, as noted earlier in this chapter. Because the number of deaths (along with death rates) increase with increasing age, age-standardized rates (as in Pappas et al., 1983) will give more weight to the older ages. Second, the analysis of Sorlie et al. (1992) involved larger numbers (cited earlier).

Another follow-up study in a national sample of adults is noteworthy because of adjustment not only for reported income for each family (in seven categories) but also for six risk factors that left a residual excess mortality of 31% in black versus white 35–54 year olds (with only one homicide among blacks) (Otten et al., 1990). The six risk factors were smoking, systolic blood pressure, blood cholesterol level, body mass index (weight divided by height), alcohol intake, and diabetes mellitus. These factors are all related to social class, although some relationships are complex. Thus, social class may operate through these factors in causal pathways involved in disease and death. Other analyses of the 1986 National Mortality Follow-back Survey have shown the importance of social class, marital status, and household size in explaining the higher death rates for blacks from some causes (including cardiovascular diseases) but not from other causes (infectious diseases, diabetes, and homicide) (Pappas, 1994; Rogers, 1992). Marital status and household size are not social class variables, although they are correlated with social class. Again, age-specific rates must be analyzed because the importance of unexplained black excesses in mortality rates varies by age group.

This book focuses on mortality. However, the final study of adults to be discussed involves morbidity. An intensive cross-sectional study of atherosclerosis in blacks and whites in three areas (11,500 whites in Washington County, MD, Minneapolis, and Forsyth County, NC, and about 4,300 blacks in Jackson, MS) provided unusually detailed information on risk factors (Diez-Roux et al., 1995). Prevalence rates for coronary heart disease (CHD), adjusted for age and gender, increased with decreasing income (obtained for each individual in the study), from more than $35,000 to less than $8,000. Rates were generally similar for blacks and whites within each income level and were lower for whites than blacks after adjustment for various CHD risk factors. The stronger association between education and CHD prevalence among whites than among blacks was regarded as consistent with the "economic effects of racism," because at similar levels of education income is lower for blacks than whites (Chapter 3). While the study involved a rather small sample of blacks living in one poor Southern community, the point is that studies of morbidity provide insights into how social class variables and race affect the risk of developing CHD. It is important to emphasize that examination of black–white differences in mortality from CHD (or other causes), as in this book (Chapter 5), brings into play factors related to survival such as access to and quality of medical care and social support (Chapter 6).

Turning to infant mortality, high black/white ratios in 1964–1966 and 1987 in national samples of live births were found within categories of maternal education from 0–8 to 16 or more years, with the highest ratios (from 1.4 to 2.3) at the higher levels of education; also, the black/white ratios increased over the time period studied (Singh and Yu, 1995). A review of black–white differences in infant mortality, including a study of low birth weight in the offspring of highly educated black parents in a national sample, suggests that the high poverty rate may not explain all of the black disadvantage in health (Hogue and Hargreaves, 1993). Unexplained black–white mortality differences could reflect (at least in part) inadequate control for black–white differences in current social class, failure to consider the effects of social class in earlier life (including childhood), intergenerational effects of social class, and the influence of other variables not considered (such as psychosocial stresses and nutrition).

In conclusion, control for social class variables does not appear to explain all of the black–white differences in mortality rates. The residual or unexplained excess among blacks may be greatest for homicides, infectious diseases, and other selected causes of death. Inclusion of various other factors correlated with (but also somewhat independent of) social class leads to further reduction in black–white disparities in mortality. Some of these other variables also could be associated with place of residence or specifically with the degree of black–white residential segregation.

Toward the Epidemiology of American Apartheid

Mortality in South Africa and America

The medical and public health literature has dealt with the effects of apartheid on the health of South African blacks. Apartheid and its health consequences may be considered as "extreme phenomena of social class" combined with a history of "colonization" and "internal colonization" associated with social caste (Susser, 1983). The "internal colonization" concept has also been used with reference to African Americans (Chapter 1). The epidemiology of American apartheid may be considered as an extension of socioeconomic epidemiology. This extension requires the perspective of sociology because of the importance of race relations and social structural issues that go beyond social class (Chapter 1).

The World Health Organization (WHO) prepared a comprehensive report titled *Apartheid and Health* (1984), although its data on the health status of South African blacks were seriously inadequate. The American Association for the Advancement of Science's *Apartheid Medicine: Health and Human Rights in South Africa* was published as a monograph, and a summary appeared as an article in the *Journal of the American Medical Association* (Nightingale et al., 1990a,b). In South Africa the concentration of poverty in predominantly black areas leads to high rates of infectious and parasitic diseases such as tuberculosis and measles among blacks. These are preventable by immunization and improvements in sanitation and living conditions.

Age-standardized mortality ratios, or comparisons of rates in one geographic area with rates for an entire country after adjusting for differences in age distribution, have been analyzed by geographic area in South Africa. Mortality ratios for various "preventable" causes of death were found to be high (in 1984–1986) for "homelands." These preventable causes included tuberculosis, cancer of the uterine cervix, rheumatic heart disease, hypertensive disease, and various respiratory diseases (and asthma, analyzed separately) (Maxwell, 1995). Under apartheid, these "homelands" were described as self-governing black territories. They were separate but hardly equal (to other areas) because they received a disproportionately low fraction of total national health expenditures. Hospitals have been segregated, and quality of care for blacks has been poor. Tertiary care in South Africa is often unequalled in the whole of Africa and is comparable to that in many areas of the United States, but a reallocation of finances to preventive and primary medical care for the "majority" (mainly blacks and "coloureds") has been advocated, along with an expanded role for teaching hospitals (Maxwell, 1995).

In the United States, medical care was also segregated in the past (Charatz-Litt, 1992) but now de facto residential segregation and the concentration of poverty in predominantly black urban areas results in differences in medical care. The lack of a personal physician and health insurance by many inner-city minority persons is a major problem in the United States. Urban teaching hospitals in America, often located in inner cities, can provide good medical care, but quality of care may differ for blacks and whites admitted to these hospitals (Chapter 6).

In the United States, as in South Africa, black–white disparities in health status persist. As in South Africa, U.S. black–white mortality differences involve mainly "preventable" deaths that could be avoided with proper preventive and health care measures. Thus, mortality differences reveal much about the quality and equality of life and medical care and are one measure of social progress. Infant mortality has been recognized as an especially sensitive indicator of the degree of social progress toward equality of opportunity and quality of environment (Yankauer, 1990; Wise and Pursley, 1992).

Infant mortality rates are expressed as the number of deaths occurring under 1 year of age per 1,000 live births during the same time period (usually one calendar year). In South Africa infant mortality rates have declined more sharply since 1960 among blacks than among whites, with the largest decline being for the "mixed" racial group (Fig. 4-1). Rates for both nonwhite groups, however, remain high, and that for "mixed race" South Africans in 1985 was about the same as the rate for U.S. blacks in 1960. Thus, although social and medical progress for blacks had been made in South Africa from 1960 to 1985, large racial disparities in infant mortality rates remain. Noteworthy is the very close approximation of the lines for South African whites and U.S. whites, indicating the effects of similar levels of social class, as well as probable similarities in quality of medical care and general environmental circumstances. In contrast to South African data on "mixed" races (Fig. 4-1), in the United States the need for data on infant mortality and other health-related variables for those who consider themselves to be of "mixed" race has only recently been recognized (Chapter 2).

The decline in infant mortality rates in the United States since the early 1960s has been attributed largely to increased survival of low-birth-weight infants, representing an effect of hospital-based high-technology neonatal care. Declines have occurred for both black and white infants, but the black–white disparity has persisted. In recent years, the black–white gap has actually increased slightly (Centers for Disease Control and Prevention, 1994) (Chapter 5).

Black infant mortality rates in some areas of the South, and also in parts of the Midwest and Northeast, have been especially high. In 1985, metropolitan counties outside urban areas in Florida had a black infant mortality rate of 29.0 in 1985 (based on 126 infant deaths). In Delaware, the rate for black infants in nonurbanized metropolitan areas reached 50.0 (based on 20 infant deaths

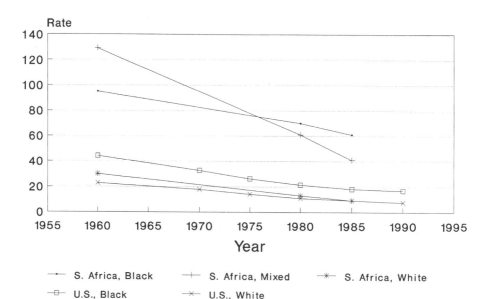

Figure 4-1. Infant mortality rates in South Africa and the United States.

in blacks (Vital Statistics of the United States, 1982–1990a). These rates are in the range of those for South African black or "mixed" race infants in 1985 (Fig. 4-1) and are similar to those in some developing countries.

Strikingly high death rates in young adult black males in the Harlem area of New York City, even higher than rates in Bangladesh, suggested that a federal "disaster area" should be declared (McCord and Freeman, 1990). As discussed later, inadequacies in medical care, related to low social class and possibly discrimination, are a major factor in these large black–white disparities in health. By way of analogy, in Bangladesh the distance to a qualified physician of Western medicine was a significant factor in infant death rates (Paul, 1991). In the United States, concentrations of extreme poverty and residential segregation are associated with lack of health insurance and lack of a regular physician, along with the frequent use of hospital emergency departments by minority persons (Chapter 5). These conditions in inner cities, disproportionately inhabited by minorities, result in poor access to diagnostic services and inadequate follow-up for treatment.

Variation in Death Rates in Large U.S. Metropolitan Areas

Background

Predictors of variation in mortality among SMSAs were examined by Kitagawa and Hauser (1973). The 201 SMSAs, now called MSAs or PMSAs (Chapter 2), included were those that had more than 5,000 total nonwhite males or females in the 1960 Census and for which more than 90% of the nonwhite males or females were black. Age-adjusted total mortality rates for all causes of death combined in "all races" and for "all nonwhites" in 1959–1961 were analyzed using 1960 Census data as "ecologic" variables at the SMSA level.

The analyses involved multiple linear regression, which was also used in this book (Chapter 5). In this statistical technique, a dependent or "outcome" variable, such as mortality rates for blacks by MSA, is selected. Several potentially useful independent variables are selected that may be associated with the dependent variables, as well as with each other. Interested readers may consult the Appendix for some notes on the technique of multiple linear regression. In Kitagawa and Hauser's analyses (1973), the variable "percent black," or the percentage of the total population of the MSA that was black in 1960, was important in predicting the age-adjusted mortality rate for all races combined. This reflects the higher mortality rates for blacks than whites (for most age groups) so that SMSAs with higher proportions of blacks in the population would tend to have higher total death rates for all races combined.

However, Kitagawa and Hauser (1973) did not include percent black as a variable in analyses of age-adjusted mortality rates by SMSA among "nonwhites" (predominantly blacks, in this study of the U.S. population in 1960). This would have provided a crude analysis of the potential influence of black–white residential segregation because percent black and the index of residential dissimilarity are strongly correlated. That is, the segregation index is higher in MSAs with large proportions of blacks due to isolating mechanisms or responses of whites to the influx of large numbers of blacks into an area (Chapter 2).

Variation in death rates: metropolitan areas used in this book
Data on social class and other variables for blacks or whites can be included in ecologic analyses of variation in death rates among large MSAs. Ecologic studies use information on the group or population level (e.g., by MSA or PMSA) rather than for specific individuals identified in a study and obtained by interviews or special surveys. Hypotheses to explain the variation in mortality rates, including the roles of social class and other factors, can be developed. The analyses in Chapter 5 include ecologic data on variation in both social class indicators for blacks and whites and the degree of black–white residential segregation among large metropolitan areas of the United States.

The study of geographic variation in black–white differences in mortality in America can identify which areas have highest and lowest mortality rates for blacks and the largest and smallest black–white differences in mortality rates. Identifying specific geographic areas that have shown marked declines or increases in the two measures over time may provide clues to understanding black–white disparities in mortality and in developing policies and interventions. The concept of "achieved minima" or the lowest rates of illness or death actually achieved in some geographic area at some time (Hahn et al., 1990) may be especially useful in planning detailed studies of factors accounting for such rates, as well as in planning interventions elsewhere.

The analyses in Chapter 5 involve MSAs and PMSAs (as defined in Chapter 2). Figure 4-2 shows the distribution of infant mortality rates for blacks in all 92 MSAs with more than 1,000 live births to black mothers in 1989–1991; white infant mortality rates are shown for these same MSAs. The difference in distributions for blacks and whites is remarkable. Blacks in many MSAs had infant mortality rates in 1989–1991 that were as high as or higher than the rates for whites in 1960 (i.e., more than 20 per 1,000 live births; Fig. 4-1).

Also included in Chapter 5 are analyses of mortality rates for adult blacks and whites; analyses focus on young and middle-aged adults, for whom the black excess in death rates compared to whites has been known for decades (as mentioned earlier). Figure 4-3 shows variations in black and white mortality rates for young adult males (15–44 years old) in 50 MSAs in 1990–1991. Because small numbers of deaths in small MSAs result in statistically unstable death rates, previous work on mortality rates has focused on all 38 MSAs with more than 1 million total population in 1980 (Polednak, 1991, 1994). For this book, mortality data were added for 12 MSAs with more than 150,000 blacks in the 1990 Census (Chapter 5).

There is more variation in mortality rates for black infants and young adults than for white infants and young adults among the MSAs examined (Figs. 4-2 and 4-3). Mortality rates for whites tend to be clustered at the lower end of the scale. A similar observation was made in an analysis of variation in mortality rates for young adults in the 342 "health areas" or districts in New York City in 1979–1981 (McCord and Freeman, 1990).

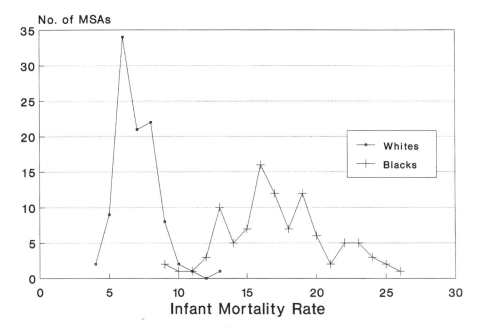

Figure 4-2. Infant mortality rates in the U.S. for blacks and whites in 92 metropolitan statistical areas (MSAs) (1989–91).

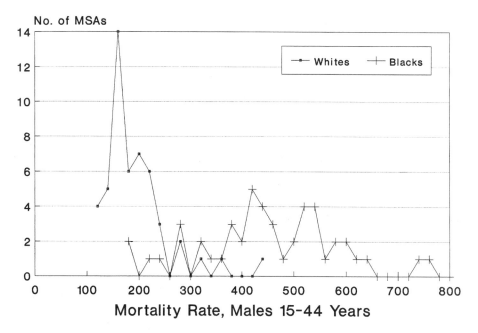

Figure 4-3. Mortality in young adults (15–44 years) in blacks and whites in 50 MSAs (1990–91).

Table 4-2. Some Characteristics of 92 MSAs with >1,000 live births to black mothers in each year during 1989–1991 used in analyses of infant mortality rates

Variable	Mean	Range
Segregation index	70	41–91
Poverty rate		
Blacks (percent)	29.0	12.2–52.8
Whites (percent)	8.1	3.5–16.2
Black/white ratio	3.8	1.6–7.1

There is also considerable variation in poverty rates for blacks and in the black/white ratios of poverty rates, as well as in the level of black–white segregation, among the MSAs used in Figures 4-2 and 4-3. Tables 4-2 and 4-3 show the averages and ranges of values for poverty rates and segregation. Although the ranges are restricted in comparison with the theoretical values that might be achieved for segregation (Chapter 2) and poverty, there is some "room" for these variables to "explain" some of the variations in death rates for blacks and in black/white ratios of death rates among the MSAs and PMSAs.

Conclusion

The roles of poverty and low social class in explaining black–white differences in mortality have been well documented in many studies in the United States since the classic work of Kitagawa and Hauser (1973) on "socioeconomic epidemiology." Studies comparing death rates of African Americans and whites suggest that a residual (unexplained) difference in mortality, or a persistence of high rates in blacks, remains after adjustment for social class variables. It has been argued that such gross statistics (Figs. 4-2 and 4-3) of black–white disparities in health-related measures should not be presented without an attempt

Table 4-3. Some characteristics of 50 MSAs used in the analysis of mortality in young adult black and white men (1990–1991)

Variable	Mean	Range
Segregation index	70	43–89
Poverty rate		
Blacks	26.9	9.7–41.3
Whites	7.6	3.5–16.2
Black/white ratio	3.7	1.4–7.1

Data for "D," or the index of residential dissimilarity between blacks and Anglos, are from Farley and Frey (1992). Other data are from the 1990 Census.

to control for black–white differences in social class. The comparisons of geographic variation of mortality rates by Kitagawa and Hauser (1973) are extended in this book to consider the effect of level of segregation (not examined by Kitagawa and Hauser). Statistical controls for social class indicators by MSA and PMSA are included in models aimed at examining the association between level of segregation in each MSA and PMSA and black death rates and in black/ white ratios of death rates in these MSAs/PMSAs (Chapter 5).

5

Segregation and Poverty in Relation to Variation in Urban Black Mortality Rates

In this chapter, some specific MSAs and PMSAs (often collectively referred to as "MSAs" in this chapter) with unusually high and low mortality rates for blacks, or black/white ratios of mortality rates, for all causes of death combined are identified. Certain ecologic data on characteristics of these MSAs are shown. Examination of these characteristics may help to explain the death rates observed.

Returning to the conceptual framework outlined in Chapter 1, the studies reviewed in this chapter consider both poverty rates and an index of segregation (the "index of dissimilarity," discussed in Chapter 2). Although education has been shown to be the most important social class variable in many studies of morbidity and mortality (Chapter 4), incomes for blacks and whites differ within the same level of education (Chapters 3 and 4). Therefore, poverty rates for black and white persons and income distributions for black and white households in each MSA and PMSA are used in the analyses in this chapter.

In some analyses, additional variables are those related to quality of life or "concentration" ("neighborhood") effects of segregation discussed in Chapter 3. In their classic study, Kitagawa and Hauser (1973) noted that the large variation in mortality rates within strata of the nonwhite population and among MSAs suggested that much of the "excess mortality" of blacks could be "reduced with increases in levels of living and lifestyles." "Lifestyle" appeared to encompass what would now be called "quality of life." If the associations between segregation and black mortality rates by MSA are affected by the inclusion of these "quality of life" (that is, neighborhood and housing) variables, then segregation may operate through these (or related) factors.

The main value of ecologic studies, using summary data for populations in political units (MSAs), is to point the way toward studies in which data are **69** obtained on individuals. Such studies would test the hypotheses generated by ecologic studies.

This chapter also refers to statistical analyses of death rates in selected large MSAs using multiple linear regression models. In these models, independent variables or "predictors" may emerge that appear to be associated with death rates after "controlling for" the effects of other variables. The models are shown in the Appendix. For readers interested in the regression models, results of tests of the "statistical significance" of regression coefficients are cited in this chapter. Also provided are the model "adjusted" R^2 (R-squared) values to indicate the success of the model in "fitting" the data (see Appendix for brief comments on regression models).

Infant Mortality

Segregation and Poverty as Predictors: Background

A study examining variation in infant death rates (all races combined) among all 50 states in 1989 included both the proportion of black persons and residential segregation indexes as "structural" variables at the state level (Bird and Bauman, 1995). In predicting variation in total infant mortality rates by state, "structural" variables, including social class and socioeconomic status, were more important than "health services" variables such as the numbers of physicians and rates of uninsured persons, delayed or no prenatal care, and state expenditures on health, hospitals, and public welfare. However, data on the association between segregation and infant mortality rates for blacks were not presented.

Kitagawa and Hauser (1973) did not include the proportion of blacks in each MSA, a variable strongly correlated with segregation (the index of dissimilarity), in their analysis of death rates for black adults by MSA in 1959–1961 (Chapter 4). However, in an even earlier study (published in a sociological journal), Yankauer (1950) examined the proportion of total live births that was nonwhite in relation to infant death rates *for nonwhites* in neighborhoods ("health areas") of New York City. First, the results (Table 5-1) showed extreme segregation in that few white live births occurred in the areas with more than 75% nonwhites, while almost half of births to "other" races (mostly blacks) occurred in these areas. Thus, the high death rates for whites in the predominantly (75%) non-white areas were based on small numbers of live births. Most striking was the trend toward rising infant death rates in "other" races as the proportion of nonwhites in the health area increased (Table 5-1).

Infant mortality, or the number of deaths per 1,000 live births, was subdivided into its two components of neonatal (less than 30 days after birth) and post-neonatal (30–364 days after birth). The association between proportion of non-whites in the health area and "other"/white ratio of death rates was slightly stronger for the postneonatal than the neonatal period (Yankauer, 1950). Postneonatal death rates are generally regarded as reflecting the overall quality of

Table 5-1. Average annual infant mortality rates (per 1,000 live births) in New York City in 1945–1947 among health areas with increasingly larger proportions of nonwhites in the population

Percent of nonwhites in area	Number of live births		Neonatal death rate		Postneonatal death rate		Infant death rate	
	White	Other	White	Other	White	Other	White	Other
<5	317,563	2,868	19.1	24.0	5.8	9.0	24.9	33.0
5–9	29,410	2,200	21.3	26.3	6.1	12.3	27.4	38.6
10–24	24,628	4,760	21.4	30.2	7.6	13.3	29.0	43.5
25–49	20,931	6,190	21.5	32.3	7.1	15.2	28.6	47.4
50–74	5,477	9,056	24.5	31.4	7.1	14.4	31.6	45.8
75+*	1,703	18,420	35.9	38.7	15.1	14.0	51.0	52.7
Total	389,712	43,494	19.6	33.7 (1.7)†	6.1	13.8 (2.3)†	25.7	47.5 (1.8)†

Modified from Yankauer (1950).

*Note: The rates for whites in the "75% + nonwhite" areas are based on a small number of live births for whites (i.e., 1,703).

† The ratios of the rates in "other" race to "white" are shown in parentheses.

the social and physical environment (Pharoah, 1979) as well as postneonatal medical care. Variation in neonatal death rates by geography and time period are related mainly to the quantity and quality of neonatal medical care.

Yankauer's work (1950) should have been groundbreaking, even though it did not consider the effect of differences in social class among the geographic areas compared. Yet, in a comprehensive 1989 report on the status of blacks in American society (Jaynes and Williams, 1989), the issue of the potential health effects of segregation was only briefly mentioned, and no studies were cited.

In a 1990 symposium on housing quality in relation to health, Struening et al. (1990) examined trends from 1969–1971 to 1985–1987 in the prevalence of low birth weight among three groups of New York City health areas defined by the percentage of the total population that was black (Table 5-2). The maximum low birth weight rate (in any health area) increased in the predominantly black areas. Although low-birth-weight rates were not examined for blacks separately, the high rates in the "90% + black" category obviously relate almost entirely to blacks. Yankauer's work (1950) was not cited.

Other studies have examined the association between mortality rates and both socioeconomic variables and segregation. In the studies reviewed in this chapter, segregation was measured by the index of dissimilarity, which measures the degree of unevenness of the residential distribution of a specific minority group across the subunits (census tracts or block groups) within an urban area (see Chapter 2 for details).

In an analysis of 176 U.S. cities, LaVeist (1989) found a positive association between the degree of black–white segregation and the infant mortality rate in 1981–1985 among blacks. This association held even when black poverty rates for each city were included in the multiple regression models. Segregation was not significantly associated with white infant mortality; the sign of the regression coefficient was negative.

Table 5-2. Total low-birth-weight rate (percent) in New York City's 338 health areas grouped by increasing proportion of blacks in the population (1970 or 1980 Census)

Percent blacks in area	1969–1971		1979–1981		1985–1987	
	Mean	Maximum	Mean	Maximum	Mean	Maximum
<10	7.0	13.2 (186)*	5.7	11.8 (155)	5.3	12.0 (155)
10–80	10.7	15.6 (133)	9.6	17.4 (160)	9.7	18.0 (160)
90+	15.1	17.6 (19)	15.2	21.5 (23)	14.9	24.7 (23)

Modified from Struening et al. (1990).
* Figures in parentheses are the numbers of "health areas" or regions in New York City.

Data for 38 Large MSAs

In a study published in 1991, Polednak did not mention the previously published work of Yankauer (1950) and LaVeist (1989). Analyses involved all 38 U.S. MSAs with more than 1 million people in 1980 (mentioned in Chapters 2 and 3). Segregation indexes were based on census tract subunits in 1980 (from Massey and Denton, 1987). The black infant mortality rate for the entire period of 1982–1986 was positively associated with segregation, even when black poverty rates, median family income, and proportion of families with a female householder were included in multiple regression models. The black–white difference in infant mortality rate was also significantly associated with the segregation index independent of the black–white difference in poverty rate. The largest black–white differences in infant mortality were in MSAs in the Northeast and North Central/Midwest regions.

Several large MSAs in California were of particular interest because of low black infant mortality rates. Due to the limited variation in white infant mortality rates (noted in Chapter 4), some of these MSAs also had small black–white differences in (or low black/white ratios of) infant mortality rates. Average annual black infant mortality rates were low for Anaheim (10.6 per 1,000 live births per year), San Jose (12.2), and Riverside (14.5) relative to Los Angeles (18.7) despite the higher poverty rate for blacks in Riverside (26.7%) than in Anaheim (15.8%) and San Jose (14.5%). The California MSAs with low black infant mortality rates and small black–white differences in infant mortality rates (Fig. 5-1) had relatively low segregation indexes (in 1980).

In most subsequent analyses in this chapter (except where otherwise indicated), the segregation indexes for various MSAs for 1980 and 1990 are based on census-block groups (averaging about 900 residents in 1980 and 560 in 1990) as subunits (Farley and Frey, 1992, 1994; Massey and Denton, 1993). Use of census-block data rather than the larger census tracts (Massey and Denton, 1987) results in higher indexes of dissimilarity that more accurately reflect the situation in the urban "neighborhoods" of each MSA (Chapter 2).

Analysis of average annual infant mortality rates in 1987–1989 in the 38 large MSAs showed the persistence of the association between degree of segregation

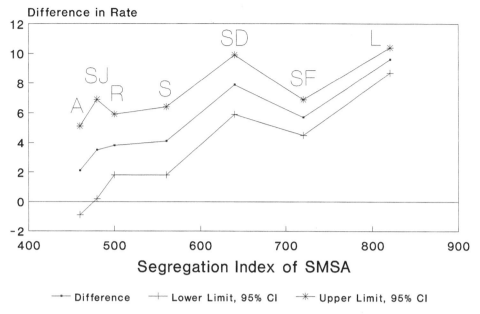

Figure 5-1. Black–white differences in infant mortality rate (per 1,000 live births per year) in California SMSAs in 1982–1986, with 95% confidence intervals (CI) of differences. A, Anaheim; SJ, San Jose; R, Riverside; S, Sacramento; SD, San Diego; SF, San Francisco; L, Los Angeles. (From Polednak, 1991.)

and infant mortality for blacks, independent of the black poverty rate, and the absence of an association for whites (Polednak, 1995). The black infant mortality rate was correlated less strongly with the black poverty rate (Pearson $r = 0.167$, $p = 0.158$) than with the segregation index ($r = 0.514$, $p < 0.001$).

In the United States as a whole, infant mortality rates declined from 1980 to 1991 for both blacks and whites, but the black/white ratio increased (Centers for Disease Control and Prevention, 1994). Variations in black and white infant mortality rates among the 38 large MSAs by time period, level of residential segregation, and geographic area have been examined (Polednak, 1996a). Deaths at less than 1 year of age for whites and blacks by MSA have been published by the National Center for Health Statistics. Numbers of live births by MSA and PMSA were published (Vital Statistics of the United States, 1982–1990) by race of the infant until 1989, when mother's race began to be used (National Center for Health Statistics, 1993, 1994). Use of the latter denominators results in slightly higher infant mortality rates for blacks. Also, higher infant death rates have been reported for biracial infants with black versus white mothers (Collins and David, 1993). However, the effect of using different denominators for "black" infant mortality rates is small, as shown in national data (National Center for Health Statistics, 1993, 1994) because of the small number of biracial births relative to births to two black parents (due to low black–white intermarriage rates, as discussed in Chapter 2).

The 38 MSAs were arranged in order of increasing level of segregation based on segregation indexes from 1980 Census data; these rankings were similar to those based on the 1990 Census. The 38 MSAs were divided into five groups or quintiles with roughly equal numbers of MSAs. The total number of infant deaths in all MSAs in a specific quintile was divided by the total number of live births in the quintiles. (The statistical reliability of infant mortality rates was examined by using 95% confidence intervals [CIs] based on the normal distribution.)

White infant mortality rates were unrelated to the segregation index (Fig. 5-2) and declined throughout the period of 1982–1991. The black infant mortality rate for most-segregated (5th quintile) MSAs declined from 1982 to 1983 but then stabilized at more than 20 per 1,000 live births. In contrast, the rate for blacks in the least-segregated MSAs was relatively low and declined from 1982 to 1985. Rates for MSAs in other quintiles of segregation were intermediate (data not shown).

In 1985, the total black infant mortality rate for the seven least-segregated MSAs was 12.5 (95% CI = 10.6–14.3) per 1,000, and the total white infant mortality rate in the 38 MSAs was 9.2 (95% CI = 9.0–9.4). Six of the seven least-segregated MSAs were located in the West (with five in California), and all seven had a black infant mortality rate of less than 15 per 1,000 live births in 1985. Three of the seven reached the Year 2000 national objective for black

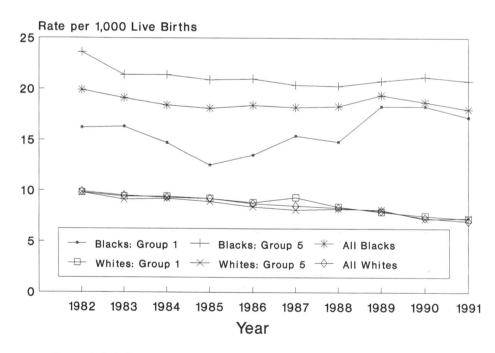

Figure 5-2. Infant mortality rate in 38 large metropolitan statistical areas in groups of MSAs with the highest and lowest black–white segregation rates, 1982–1991. (From Polednak, 1996a.)

infant mortality (U.S. Public Health Service, 1991) of 11 per 1,000. These MSAs were San Antonio, San Jose, and Sacramento), The other four MSAs were Phoenix, Riverside, San Diego, and Anaheim. The infant mortality rate for blacks (but not whites) in the least-segregated MSAs increased sharply after 1985 (Fig. 5-2).

In 1982–1986, as noted earlier, the segregation index in 1980 (based on census tract units) was a significant predictor of the black infant mortality rate in 1982–1986, when the black poverty rate of each MSA was included in a multiple linear regression model (Polednak, 1991). In a similar model for 1989–1991, however, the 1990 segregation index did not reach statistical significance as an independent variable ($t = 1.54$, $p = 0.134$) in predicting the black infant mortality rate in the 38 MSAs; the model R^2 was only 0.019. This finding for 1989–1991 is consistent with the decline in the magnitude of the difference in black infant mortality rate between the highest and lowest quintiles of segregation (Fig. 5-2). Segregation index in 1990 and black poverty rate in 1990 were highly correlated (Pearson $r = 0.631$), but not strongly enough to consider discarding a variable.

The rate of unmarried black mothers by MSA in 1990, or the midpoint of the 1989–1991 time interval, was highly correlated with the segregation index ($r = 0.747$). When the rate of black unmarried mothers was added to the regression model, along with the segregation index and the black poverty rate, it was the only variable associated with the black infant mortality rate ($t = 3.45$). (The model adjusted R^2 was 0.252).

In the analyses discussed thus far, all of the least-segregated MSAs and PMSAs were located in the West, mostly in California, except for one in Texas. The next analyses were intended to examine recent changes in black infant mortality rates in a larger number of individual MSAs and PMSAs

Data for Larger Numbers of MSAs

Eighty-eight MSAs in 1991 versus 1985

There were 88 MSAs and PMSAs with more than 1,000 "black" live births in 1985. They were grouped by level of segregation (in 1980) and census-defined geographic regions and divisions, and black and white infant mortality rates were calculated for 1985 and 1991. These 88 MSAs included about 75% of all births to black mothers in the United States in 1991. MSAs in the lowest quintile of segregation had segregation indexes of 65 or lower, and the highest quintile included segregation indexes of 82 or higher. All MSAs in the lowest (but none in the highest) quintile of segregation in 1985 and 1991 were located either in the western region, including California (Riverside, Sacramento, San Diego, and San Jose MSAs), or the southern region. Most of the MSAs in the 5th (or highest) quintile were located in the Middle Atlantic and East North Central divisions, with a few in the South Atlantic division. "South" (Table 5-3) refers to the South Atlantic, East South Central, and West South Central divisions combined. Definitions of a few MSAs, or PMSAs and New England County MAs (NECMAs), changed over time; for these analyses, for example,

Table 5-3. Black infant mortality rates (IMRs) in 1985 and 1991 for the least- and most-segregated of 88 U.S. MSAs*

Area or group	IMR (and 95% CI)	1980 Segregation index	1980 Poverty (Percent)	IMR (and 95% CI)	1990 Segregation index	1990 Poverty (Percent)
	1985			**1991**		
BLACKS IN LEAST-SEGREGATED MSAs						
West (7)	12.8 (11.0–14.9)	58	21	17.6 (15.7–19.8)	52	22
South (11)	19.3 (17.6–21.1)	60	31	16.8 (15.4–18.3)	57	27
Total (18)	17.0 (15.7–18.4)	59	27	17.1 (16.0–18.3)	55	25
BLACKS IN MOST-SEGREGATED MSAs						
Total (16)	20.7 (19.9–21.5)	86	30	20.2 (19.5–20.9)	82	32
ALL 88 MSAs						
Blacks (88)	18.4 (18.0–18.8)	74	29	17.8 (17.4–18.2)	70	29
Whites (88)	9.3 (9.1–9.5)	74	8	7.1 (7.0–7.2)	70	8

Modified from Polednak (1996a).

Denominators of infant mortality rates for 1985 were live births in 1985 based on race of infant. Denominators for 1991 were live births in 1991 based on race of mother.

"Least segregated" refers to a segregation index of 65 or lower (range, 43–65) based on the 1980 Census data. "Most segregated" refers to a segregation index of 82 or higher (range, 82–91).

In the Bureau of the Census' geographic areas, the "West" includes states west of Texas, North Dakota, South Dakota, Nebraska, and Kansas. The "South" includes the South Atlantic (West Virginia, Maryland, Delaware, Washington, DC, Virginia, North Carolina, South Carolina, Georgia, and Florida), East South Central (Kentucky, Tennessee, Mississippi, and Alabama) and West South Central (Texas, Oklahoma, Arkansas, and Louisiana) divisions.

* All had more than 1,000 "black" live births in 1985.

Dallas was combined with Fort Worth, TX, and San Francisco with Oakland, CA, in 1991 for compatibility with 1985.

For the least-segregated MSAs, western (but not southern) MSAs had a low total black infant mortality rate in 1985 (Table 5-3). These western MSAs were the same as those involved in the earlier analyses (Fig. 5-2) except that Anaheim (with less than 1,000 black births per year) was excluded while Las Vegas and Tacoma were added. In 1985, all of these MSAs had black infant mortality rates less than 15 per 1,000 live births except for Tacoma (at 15.1 per 1,000). By 1991, the advantage for the West had disappeared. This was due to an increase for western MSAs and a decrease for southern MSAs. Of the western MSAs only Tacoma (12.9) and San Diego (14.0) had a black rate of less than 15 in 1991.

The difference in the total black infant mortality rate between the MSAs in the lowest and highest quintiles of segregation was smaller in 1991 than in 1985

(Table 5-3) (as in Fig. 5-2). This was due in part to the fact that the black infant mortality rate for the least-segregated southern MSAs in 1991 was not as low as that reached by the western MSAs in 1985. Rates of unwed mothers (per 1,000 live births for each race) were higher for blacks than for whites and higher for blacks in the most-segregated than the least segregated MSAs among the 88 MSAs studied (Table 5-4).

The black/white ratio of infant mortality rates in the 88 MSAs increased from 2.0 in 1985 to 2.5 in 1991. These results include any effect (albeit small) of the temporal change in the definition of the denominator for black rates (mentioned above). That is, starting in 1989, the denominators for "black" infant mortality rates were the numbers of live births to black mothers.

Achieved minimum rates in 1985 and 1991
Of major interest were MSAs where black infants had achieved low infant mortality rates. Demonstration of such "achieved minimum" death rates "at some time and place" (Hahn et al., 1990) should be useful in planning intensive studies to search for explanations. Such studies could lead to the development of interventions to reduce black infant mortality rates in other geographic areas or to the promotion and expansion of some existing programs.

In 1985, three of the five MSAs with black rates of about 11 per 1,000 or lower were located in the West, and all five were in the lowest quintile of segregation. As mentioned earlier, the 11.0 figure is the Year 2000 national objective for blacks (U.S. Public Health Service, 1991). However, three of the four MSAs with black infant mortality rates as low as about 11 per 1,000 in 1991 were in the South, and only one was in the lowest quintile of segregation (Table 5-5). Only the rate for the Boston area in 1991 was based on more than 50 infant deaths (i.e., 103) and more than 5,000 live births; the latter number was

Table 5-4. Change in rate of live births to unwed mothers, 1985 to 1991*

Area or group	Unwed mothers (1985)	Unwed mothers (1991)	Percent change
BLACKS IN LEAST-SEGREGATED MSAs			
West (7)	490	587	+20
South (11)	487	577	+24
Total (18)	488	581	+19
BLACKS IN MOST-SEGREGATED MSAs			
Total (16)	668	740	+11
All 88 MSAs			
Blacks (88)	593	672	+13
Whites (88)	131	192	+47

*Rates are per 1,000 live births for each group.

considered "statistically reliable" (National Center for Health Statistics, 1993, 1994). The low rate in the Boston area in 1991 represented a considerable decline from the rate of 21.5 per 1,000 in 1985. (Statistically, the other black infant mortality rates in Table 5-5 had wide 95% CIs on the basis of either the Poisson or normal distribution, but the upper limit was less than 14 for three of the four rates for 1991 in Table 5-5.)

With regard to regional patterns among all MSAs with more than 1,000 black live births in 1985, MSAs in the West and West–Southwest had the lowest black infant mortality rate, while in 1991 among 103 MSAs with more than 1,000 live births to black mothers (Table 5-6) the New England area had the lowest black infant mortality rate because of the low black rate in the Boston area (Table 5-5). These data show that a regional shift occurred between 1985 and 1991 in the MSAs with the lowest (or "achieved minimum") black infant mortality rates.

Data for 92 MSAs in 1989–1991
In view of the small denominators involved in rates for a single year, all MSAs with more than 1,000 live births to black mothers in *each* year from 1989 to 1991 were analyzed. None of these 92 MSAs (listed in Appendix Table A-1) had a rate for blacks of 11 or lower in 1989–1991. Of the six MSAs with rates less than 14 per 1,000 live births per year, Boston was lowest; the other five were in the South (i.e., Killeen and Austin, TX, Chattanooga, TN, Columbia, SC, and Jackson, MS). These data indicate that caution should be exercised when using black infant mortality rate data for a single year (as done for 1985 and 1991) due to statistical unreliability.

When all 92 MSAs were included in a regression model, the segregation

Table 5-5. MSAs with the lowest black infant mortality rates (11 per 1,000 live births or lower) in 1985 and 1991*

MSA	Rate	Segregation index
1985		
Fayetteville, NC	10.9	43
Las Vegas, NV	11.3	64
Sacramento, CA	11.3	60
San Antonio, TX	10.3	65
San Jose, CA	8.6	48
1991		
Boston, MA	11.1	70
Greenville, SC	10.0	63
Huntsville, AL	10.7	64
Killeen, TX	8.5	45

*Denominators for 1985 were live births based on race of infant; denominators for 1991 were live births based on race of mother.

Table 5-6. Infant mortality rates in 1985 and 1991 for blacks in MSAs with >1,000 black live births in selected geographic areas in the United States

Area*	1985			1991			
	Rate	Number of MSAs	Mean segregation index	Rate	Number of MSAs	Mean segregation index	Mean poverty
West	17.8	12	65	16.6	12	58	22
South	18.3	47	72	16.9	52	66	31
WSC	16.9	(13)	73	15.3	(15)	66	34
Mid-Atlantic and ENC	18.6	21	81	19.0	30	78	29
New England	21.5	4	73	13.4	5	70	21
All blacks	18.4 (18.0–18.8)†	88	74	17.7 (17.4–18.1)†	103	69	29
All whites	9.3	88	74	7.1	103	69	8

*WSC, West South Central (Oklahoma, Arkansas, Louisiana, and Texas). ENC, East North Central (Wisconsin, Michigan, Illinois, Indiana, and Ohio). The Mid-Atlantic division of the Northeast region includes New York, Pennsylvania, and New Jersey. The New England division of the Northeast region includes all states in the Northeast except those in the Mid-Atlantic division.
† 95% confidence interval.

index (and not the black poverty rate) was a significant predictor of the black infant mortality rate (Appendix Table A-2). The inclusion of southern MSAs with relatively low black infant mortality rates and relatively low segregation indexes contributed to the greater importance of the segregation index in this model than in the model (mentioned above) for black infant mortality rates in 38 large MSAs in 1989–1991. In another model (not shown), the rate of unmarried black mothers was the only statistically significant predictor ($t = 2.96, p = .004$) of black infant mortality rates in 1989–1991 (model $R^2 = 0.133$).

Of the 19 MSAs with black rates of more than 20 per 1,000 live births per year in 1989–1991, 13 were located in the Mid-Atlantic and East North Central divisions as defined by the Bureau of the Census (Table 5-7), which contain several hypersegregated MSAs. The four MSAs with a lower 95% CI of more than 20 (all having a total of >10,000 live births to black mothers in 1989–1991) were Chicago (24.5; 23.5–25.5), Pittsburgh (24.1; 21.3–26.9), Nassau and Suffolk Counties, NY (23.2; 20.5–25.9), and Detroit (22.4; 21.3–23.6). All four MSAs and PMSAs had a segregation index above 75 (Table 5-7).

Differences in black infant mortality rates between western and southern MSAs in the lowest quintile of segregation occurred in 1985 and 1991 despite virtually identical mean rates of unmarried black mothers (Table 5-4). Also, the infant mortality rate declined after 1985 for whites but not blacks, while the proportional increase in the rate of unmarried mothers was larger for whites. A similar trend in rates of unwed mothers has occurred in the United States. Higher rates of unwed black mothers in highly segregated urban areas (Mayer and Jencks, 1989) or some associated variables (such as short interpregnancy intervals) (Rawlings et al., 1995) not included in the regression models could have contributed to the persistence of high black infant mortality rates in the

Table 5-7. MSAs with black infant mortality rates in 1989–1991 higher than 20 per 1,000 live births*

Area MSA	Number of deaths	Total births	Rate	95% CI	Black poverty	Segregation index	Region
Albany, GA	75	3,481	21.6	16.7–26.5	41	70	5
Atlantic City	78	3,274	23.8	18.6–29.1	21	72	2
Chicago	2,351	95,882	24.5	23.5–25.5	30	87	3
Cleveland	519	24,812	20.9	19.1–22.7	31	86	3
Detroit	1,514	67,500	22.4	21.3–23.6	33	89	3
Flint	142	6,600	21.5	18.0–25.0	37	84	3
Indianapolis	243	11,783	20.6	18.1–23.2	26	80	3
Macon, GA	141	6,297	22.4	18.7–26.1	33	60	5
Minneapolis	174	7,649	22.8	19.4–26.1	37	65	4
Nassau and Suffolk Counties, NY	284	12,236	23.2	20.5–25.9	12	79	2
Norfolk	509	24,057	21.2	19.3–23.0	25	57	5
Philadelphia	1,338	64,951	20.6	19.5–21.7	26	82	2
Pittsburgh	280	11,601	24.1	21.3–26.9	36	75	2
Rochester, NY	167	8,072	20.7	17.6–23.8	32	70	2
Syracuse	66	3,279	20.1	15.3–24.9	36	76	2
Trenton	96	4,417	21.7	17.4–26.0	20	76	2
Washington, DC	1,350	67,075	20.1	19.1–21.2	13	68	5
Wilmington, DE	125	5,852	21.4	17.7–25.1	21	64	5
Youngstown	78	3,836	20.3	15.9–24.8	41	79	3

The states in which certain MSAs are located are indicated for selected MSAs to avoid confusion with other MSAs; full titles for all MSAs are listed in the Appendix.
*The 95% confidence intervals on rates are based on the normal approximation.

most-segregated MSAs in 1982–1991 (Fig. 5-2; Table 5-7), as discussed in Chapter 6. The persistently high black infant mortality rates in hypersegregated MSAs emphasize the lack of recent social progress for blacks (Yankauer, 1990).

High black mortality rates (more than 20 per 1,000 live births per year) involved mainly MSAs and PMSAs in the Mid-Atlantic and East North Central regions (regions 2 and 3 in Table 5-7), which include several large hypersegregated MSAs (Massey and Denton, 1993). These two regions included 17 of the 21 most-segregated MSAs and PMSAs. The high black infant mortality rates for the 30 MSAs and PMSAs in these two regions had the effect of diluting the declines (from 1985) for blacks in MSAs in other regions. There was also a large decline in total infant mortality rate for whites for all the MSAs in this study, as also found in the United States as a whole (National Center for Health Statistics, 1994). As a result of these trends, the black/white ratio of infant death rates was higher in 1991 than in 1985 in the MSAs studied here (Table 5-3). This change over time was also apparent in the United States as a whole (Centers for Disease Control and Prevention, 1994; National Center for Health Statistics, 1994).

The black/white ratio of poverty rates by MSA was a statistically significant predictor of the black/white infant death rate in 92 MSAs in 1989–1991 ($t =$

2.69, $p = 0.009$), but the segregation index was not a predictor ($t = 0.08$, $p = 0.938$). Very high black/white poverty ratios were evident for many hypersegregated MSAs, which also had high black infant mortality rates and high black/white ratios of infant mortality rates. As noted earlier, a low black/white ratio of infant mortality rates can be due to a high rate for whites as well as a low rate for blacks. Some MSAs in the South had high white infant mortality rates due to relatively high poverty rates for whites in the South (higher than in other regions) and to the fact that white poverty rate was a significant predictor of white infant mortality rate by MSA and PMSA. Hence, the relatively low black/white ratios of infant mortality rates in some southern MSAs and PMSAs may explain the finding that segregation was not a predictor of the black/white ratio of infant mortality rates.

Quality of Housing and Neighborhood as Predictors

The finding of an association (albeit limited) between level of segregation and black infant mortality rates in 1989–1991 due mainly to high rates in hypersegregated MSAs could reflect many factors that are independent of variation in black poverty rates. Among these factors is a constellation of factors that might be called "quality of life" (Yankauer, 1950), including the "quality" of housing and the neighborhood. Data on housing and neighborhood quality for housing units with black householder were obtained from *Current Housing Reports,* which are supplements to the American Housing Survey for selected metropolitan areas that is conducted by the U.S. Bureau of the Census. These supplements provide more detailed information than that published in the decennial census reports, although only a limited number of MSAs are surveyed each year. The MSAs included in analyses of mortality in black infants were those surveyed in the period from 1988 to 1992 or around the time of the 1990 Census and the time period (1989–1991) for which black infant mortality rates were analyzed.

Housing and neighborhood quality were each rated on a scale from 1 (for worst) to 10 (for best or highest quality) by residents or neighbors; independent observers were not used. Also, small samples of houses were involved in each large geographic area. Therefore, the results may not be representative of each entire MSA. Data were available only for 34 of the 92 MSAs used in the analysis of infant mortality rates for 1989–1991. These MSAs are shown in Appendix Table A-3, along with data on housing and neighborhood quality for blacks only. The proportion of houses with 1.01 or more persons per room, a variable also used by Kitagawa and Hauser (1973) in their analyses of death rates for 1960, was low in all MSAs, and variation was not large. The proportion of respondents who rated their neighborhoods as relatively poor quality (i.e., 1–4 on the scale of 1–10) varied from 2% to 22%, while the proportion who rated their houses as below average showed less variation.

For these 34 MSAs, prediction of black infant mortality rates was poor (results not shown). Neither the black poverty rate nor the segregation index was an important predictor. Five variables included in a regression model were black poverty rate, segregation index, proportion of respondents giving a below-average rating for neighborhood quality and housing quality, and proportion of households with more than one person per room (1.01 + persons per room). Only the neighborhood quality variable was a marginal predictor ($t = 1.61, p = 0.119$) of the black infant death rate in 34 MSAs. This represents an effect independent of the association between neighborhood quality and the segregation index, because the latter was also included in the model.

Crime rates are an aspect of quality of neighborhood. The total rate (all races combined) of homicide and non-negligent manslaughter per 100,000 population in 1990 by MSA was available for 81 of the 92 MSAs (Federal Bureau of Investigation, 1991). It was hypothesized that the homicide rate might be an indicator of overall quality of the environment and could be associated with various stresses that might adversely affect pregnancy outcome. However, total homicide rate by MSA was not strongly correlated with the segregation index ($r = 0.084$) and was negatively rather than positively correlated with black infant mortality rate ($r = -0.148$) among the 81 MSAs (data not shown). This was explained in part by very high homicide rates (>19 per 100,000 per year) in certain southern MSAs (with relatively low black infant mortality rates), including Birmingham, Jacksonville, Memphis, New Orleans, Richmond, VA, and Shreveport, LA. Future studies should examine homicide rates separately for blacks and whites at both the census tract and block level (see Chapter 6).

Conclusion

In comparison with analyses of infant mortality rates for the early to middle 1980s, the segregation index had become less important in predicting variation in black infant mortality rates among larger MSAs by 1989–1991. This was not due to any improvement in the situation for blacks, because there was no decline in infant mortality rates in hypersegregated ares. Rather, the advantage in black infant mortality rate for certain MSAs in the West with relatively low levels of segregation (especially by 1985) was lost by 1991. The very low black infant mortality rates reached by groups of least-segregated western MSAs in 1985 were not achieved by southern MSAs in 1991.

However, in 1989–1991 there was still a difference in the black infant mortality rates between MSAs and PMSAs in the least- and most-segregated groups. Moreover, a consistent finding over time has been the high black infant mortality rates for a group of hypersegregated MSAs located mainly in parts of the Northeast (excluding New England) and the Midwest. Further studies are needed, involving additional variables (Chapter 6). In all studies, the black poverty rate by MSA was not a statistically significant predictor of black infant mortality rates, when segregation index was included in regression models (La Veist, 1989; Polednak, 1991).

Analysis of time trends in black infant mortality rates by geographic area and geographic variation in these rates in recent years (1989–1991) suggested that factors other than poverty and segregation had become important in explaining this variation. The delineation of these factors should be a major priority for public health research. Studies of MSAs with "achieved minimum" death rates (Hahn et al., 1990) may provide clues regarding possible structural and health-care delivery factors (not related to segregation) that are important in influencing black infant mortality rates.

Studies of time trends in black infant mortality rates in MSAs that differ in historical levels of segregation might be rewarding. In 1911–1915 in eight U.S. cities in the North and North Central regions, within groups defined by father's income, blacks had infant mortality rates only about 10% higher than native whites. Infants of low-income mothers not employed outside the home showed no disadvantage to blacks (Ewbank, 1987). Although most of the blacks lived in a single area (Baltimore), this finding is of interest in relation to studies in later years, after increases in black–white residential segregation had occurred in Baltimore. Additional studies are needed of historical trends in black–white differences in infant mortality, after adjusting for social class, in different geographic areas with differing time trends in black–white residential segregation.

Adult Mortality

McCord and Freeman (1990) showed that the highest mortality rates in New York City in 1979–1981, especially among young adults, were in areas with a black majority population. Variation in the black–white disparity in social class was not considered. Nevertheless, the findings indicated a major challenge to public health and social policy. Consistent with the literature in socioeconomic epidemiology (Chapter 4, Table 4-1), the highest black/white ratios of mortality rates in New York City were for young and middle-aged adults (25–34-year-old women and 35–44-year-old men) in 1979–1981. Analyses of death rates for ages under 65 years in New York City's 342 health areas with a total population of more than 3,000 disclosed that 53 of the 54 areas with at least twice the number of deaths than expected on the basis of national death rates for whites had populations in which blacks comprised the majority. Mortality rates for predominantly white areas were narrowly clustered at levels close to the national rates for whites, while predominantly black or Hispanic areas had mortality ratios ranging from 0.59 to 3.95. This pattern was mentioned in Chapter 4 with reference to MSAs.

Harlem health areas had mortality ratios of 2.16 to 3.95, or death rates about two to four times those for U.S. whites, but variation in black death rates by health area was not analyzed according to variation in level of segregation and black poverty rate. Studies that have included these variables are now reviewed.

Segregation and Poverty as Predictors:
Young Adults (15–44 Years Old)

Data for 38 MSAs in 1982–1986
The degree of black–white segregation in 1980 has been shown to be associated with the black/white ratio of age-adjusted total death rates in 1982–86 for ages

15–44 years (Polednak, 1993) in the same 38 large MSAs used in the studies of infant mortality. The trend in Figure 5-3 is due to the effects of the positive association between segregation and low social class in black, as well as to the effect of segregation independent of differences in social class. However, in multiple regression analyses, the positive association between segregation and mortality was largely limited to blacks. The segregation index was a significant predictor of black/white mortality ratio when the black/white ratio of poverty rates was included in the regression model (Appendix Table A-4). Also, the MSAs with the highest black/white mortality ratios (e.g., Detroit, Newark, and St. Louis) were in the Northeast and North Central/Midwest regions and had some of the highest segregation ratios (Fig. 5-3) but not the highest black/white ratios of poverty rates.

Because of the limitations of poverty rate as an indicator of social class (Chapter 3), regression models also used other social class measures by MSA. Median household income in 1989 (as reported in the 1990 Census) for blacks and whites in each MSA was strongly correlated with the poverty rate (Pearson r = 0.90 or greater), indicating "multicolinearity." Because poverty rates were better predictors in regression models, results using median household income are not shown. Other models used the proportions of black and white house-

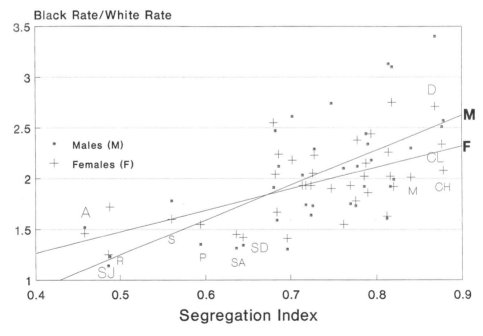

Figure 5-3. Black/white ratio of age-standardized mortality rates (1982–1986) in 38 large MSAs by segregation index of MSA. A, Anaheim, CA; CH, Chicago, IL; CL, Cleveland, OH; D, Detroit, MI; M, Minneapolis, MN; P, Phoenix, AR; R, Riverside, CA; S, Sacramento, CA; SA, San Antonio, TX; SD, San Diego, CA; SJ, San Jose, CA. (From Polednak, 1995).

holds with incomes of less than $10,000 instead of poverty rates. Again, these models did not result in a prediction of mortality rates for black males 15–44 years old that was better than that obtained by using poverty rates (Polednak, 1993).

Data for 50 MSAs in 1990–1991
The number of MSAs and PMSAs (320 in 1991) that can be included in statistically meaningful analyses of mortality in adults is smaller than that for infant mortality, because the latter rates are higher than rates for young adults and are statistically more reliable. While infant mortality rates are usually expressed per 1,000 (live births), rates per 100,000 population are often used for adults. For many MSAs, the number of deaths per year among young black adults (by gender) is less than five per age group under 35 years.

The analyses of mortality rates in 1990–1991 for black and white adults presented in this book include all 38 MSAs with more than 1 million total population in 1980 (described earlier) and 12 additional MSAs with at least 150,000 total black population in 1990, as mentioned in Chapter 4 (see Fig. 4-3). Analyses of the 50 MSAs were limited to 1990–1991. Data for 1989 were excluded because of changes in the definitions of some MSAs between 1989 and 1990. In 1980 Census reports, San Francisco and Oakland comprised a single MSA, but in 1990 they were separated. Because of the smaller population size for San Francisco, only Oakland was used for the analyses of adults.

Age-standardized rates for ages 15–44 years were calculated using the "direct" method of standardization. This involves multiplying the age-specific rates for each race by the proportions of each age group among all U.S. residents 15–25, 25–34, and 35–44 years old in 1990; the sum of these products is the age-standardized rate. All 50 MSAs are listed in Appendix Table A-5, with segregation indexes and poverty rates for 1990. Age-standardized death rates for black men 15–44 years of age for each of these 50 MSAs are shown in Figure 5-4, in relation to the segregation index in 1990 (from Farley and Frey, 1992, 1994). Figure 5-4 shows the same pattern as previously indicated for 1982-86 (Figure 5-3). In Figure 5-4 the death rate for black men rather than the black/white ratio of death rates (Fig. 5-3) was used; as noted earlier (Chapter 4), there was much more variation in death rates for blacks than for whites among the MSAs. Although there is considerable "scatter" in the data points in Figure 5-4, there is a clear positive association between segregation and the age-standardized mortality rate for black men 15–44 years old.

The 50 MSAs were arranged in order of increasing level of segregation and divided into four groups of roughly equal numbers (quartiles) of MSAs (Table 5-8). The average (mean) age-standardized death rate for black men 15–44 years of age increased across the quartiles defined by segregation. There was also an increase in the mean black poverty rate, but the increase was slight from the second to the third quartile, with no increase from the third to the fourth. The total number of deaths among black men in this age group among the 50 MSAs in 1990–1991 was 44,031 (77.7% of all 56,686 deaths in the 320 MSAs of the United States in the same age group in 1990–1991).

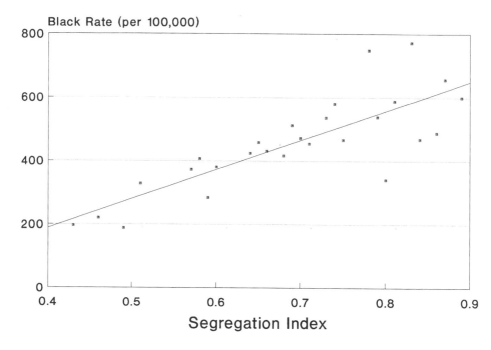

Figure 5-4. Mortality rates for black males 15–44 years old (age-standardized rate) by segregation index in 50 MSAs, 1990–1991. For MSAs with the same segregation index, the average of the death rates was used; thus, less than 50 values are plotted.

The segregation index was correlated with the black poverty rate by MSA ($r = 0.495$), but not strongly enough to present a problem for the regression analysis. The age-standardized death rate (15–44 years) for black men was more strongly correlated with the segregation index ($r = 0.676$) than with the black poverty rate ($r = .0191$) by MSA. In multiple regression analyses using the 50 MSAs, in each age group (15–24, 25–34, and 35–44 years) the segregation index was a statistically significant predictor of the age-specific black mortality rate and the black/white ratio of age-specific mortality rates (Appendix Table A-6). The segregation index was a statistically significant predictor of the age-standardized rate (ages 15–44 years) as expected from the findings for each age group when analyzed separately. The adjusted R^2 values for age-standardized black mortality rate and the black/white mortality ratio of mortality rates indicated that about 50% of the variation in these dependent variables (mortality rates) across the 50 MSAs was explained by the models. These proportions are considerable for analyses involving such a limited number of independent variables in the models.

As was done previously (Polednak, 1993), analyses were conducted using indicators of income or socioeconomic status other than the poverty rate. The proportion of black households with an income of less than $10,000 was very highly correlated with the black poverty rate (Pearson $r = 0.95$), indicating

Table 5-8. Mean age-standardized death rates (ASRs) per 100,000 (per year) for black men 15–44 years old in 1990–1991 in 50 MSAs divided into quartiles defined by increasing level of segregation

Segregation index		Number of MSAs	Black poverty mean	Black Males			White ASR mean
Range	Mean			Total number	Number of deaths	ASR mean	
43–64	54.9	12	21.9	509,607	3,167	329	196
	(6.2)*		(6.1)			(87)	(51)
65–70	67.1	12	25.2	875,733	8,403	456	202
	(1.8)		(6.0)			(82)	(49)
71–76	73.9	13	30.9	1,149,339	11,789	495	219
	(1.7)		(6.5)			(90)	(58)
78–89	82.5	13	29.1	1,716,410	20,672	542	191
	(3.4)		(7.5)			(135)	(80)

*Standard deviations of the distributions are in parentheses.

"multicolinearity" or a correlation too high for both to be used as independent variables in the same regression model. Substitution of this low-income variable for the poverty rate had no effect on the association between the age-standardized mortality rate (ages 15–44 years) and the segregation index. While the segregation index and the black poverty rate were strongly correlated (Pearson $r = 0.495$), the correlation coefficient was not high enough to indicate "multicolinearity" or to consider removing one of these two independent variables. The black mortality rate was more strongly correlated with the segregation index ($r = 0.640$) than with the black poverty rate ($r = 0.189$) by MSA. (Stepwise regression is often used when two independent variables or "predictors" are correlated. In a forward stepwise regression model, the segregation index was the only variable selected; black poverty rate and proportion of black households with incomes less than $10,000 by MSA were not selected because p was greater than 0.05.)

In an analysis of the age-standardized death rate for black males 15–44 years old, the proportion of blacks with incomes of less than 50% of the poverty level was not a significant predictor, while the segregation index was still significant ($t = 5.50$, $p < 0.01$) (data not shown).

Separate regression models were done within subgroups of MSAs defined by the black poverty rate. The association between the segregation index and the age-standardized mortality rate in black males (ages 15–44 years) was stronger within the 18 MSAs with lower rates of black poverty (less than 25%) than within the remaining 32 MSAs (black poverty rates 25% or greater). However, the segregation index was a statistically significant predictor within both groups of MSAs. The numbers of MSAs involved in these analyses were small, and the range of the segregation index was limited within the MSAs with the highest black poverty rates.

For women 15–44 years old, the age-standardized death rate for blacks was more strongly correlated with the segregation index ($r = 0.563$) than with the black poverty rate ($r = 0.133$), as also found for black men. The results of multiple regression for black women (Appendix Table A-7) were similar to those for black men in 1990–1991. The segregation index was a statistically significant predictor of the age-standardized death rate for black women and of the black/white ratio of death rates for women 15–44 years old.

Rates in black men 15–44 years old by MSA
MSAs with the lowest and highest age-standardized death rates (ages 15–44 years) for black men are listed in Table 5-9); mortality rates for all 50 MSAs are shown in Appendix Table A-8. Black/white poverty ratios (from the 1990 Census) and black–white segregation indexes were relatively low for several MSAs in the West, mainly in California. As found for 1982–1986 (described earlier), in 1990–1991 several MSAs in the West and Southwest had black/white mortality ratios for ages 15–44 years that were less than 1.5 (Table 5-9). As noted in Chapter 2, the segregation indexes for these MSAs were relatively low, although the lowest were greater than 45 (Appendix Table A-5). Noteworthy is Anaheim–Santa Ana, CA, with a black/white ratio of age-standardized death rates for men (15–44 years) of only 0.80 (Table 5-9). Relatively low black/white ratios were also evident for other California MSAs (Riverside, San Diego, and San Jose), along with Denver and Phoenix. Such low rates for blacks (and

Table 5-9. Black/white ratios of mortality rates for young adult males and age-standardized mortality rates (ages 15–44 years) in selected MSAs and PMSAs, 1990–1991

MSA*	Black/white ratios of age-specific rates			Age-standardized rates (ASRs)			Segregation index	Black poverty (percent)
	15–24	25–34	35–44	Black	White	Ratio		
LOWEST BLACK ASRs (<300)								
Anaheim	1.05	.49	1.10	195.6	245.0	.80	43	10
Denver	1.23	1.51	1.35	297.2	216.0	1.38	66	25
Riverside	1.32	1.43	1.18	188.8	145.3	1.30	49	20
San Diego	1.14	.97	1.35	282.3	238.5	1.18	59	21
San Jose	1.57	.93	1.40	223.0	174.2	1.28	45	13
HIGHEST BLACK ASRs (>550)								
Baltimore	2.21	4.01	4.09	593.0	160.8	3.69	75	23
Chicago	2.81	3.65	3.28	656.9	199.1	3.30	87	30
Detroit	3.68	3.59	3.86	600.8	161.1	3.73	89	33
Los Angeles	1.47	1.58	1.61	566.8	362.0	1.57	71	21
Miami	2.63	2.23	1.97	604.9	281.4	2.15	75	30
New Orleans	2.77	2.85	2.01	636.6	259.7	2.45	74	41
New York, NY	1.69	1.59	1.72	746.6	446.8	1.67	78	25
Newark	2.57	4.28	5.61	772.3	166.4	4.64	83	25
Jacksonville	2.91	2.85	2.63	559.7	203.2	2.75	65	29
Oakland	2.96	2.56	2.46	550.2	211.7	2.60	69	21

*For data on all 50 MSAs and PMSAs, see Appendix. Age-standardized rates are per 100,000 per year.

low black/white ratios of rates) require further study, because the explanation (if not due to chance) could provide important clues for interventions elsewhere.

Low black/white ratios of death rates may be due to low black death rates or to high white death rates, as noted earlier. Low black/white ratios in Los Angeles and New York City were due to high mortality rates in whites (relative to rates for whites in other MSAs) and not to low rates for blacks (Table 5-8). None of the MSAs in the South with more than 150,000 blacks in the population in 1990 had black/white ratios of death rates less than 2.0 (see Appendix Table A-8).

The highest black/white ratios of age-standardized death rates for men tended to occur in the older MSAs and PMSAs of the Northeast and Midwest, due to high death rates for blacks. Age-standardized rates were above 600 per 100,000 per year for Chicago, Detroit, New York, and Newark; because of the large numbers of black deaths involved, standard errors for these death rates were relatively small (data not shown). The highest black death rate was for Newark, and the relatively low rate for whites resulted in a high black/white ratio (i.e., 4.64; Table 5-9). The total homicide rate for Newark, for all races combined, was not high relative to those in other MSAs (see later). The high death rate for young-adult blacks is interesting historically. In *Newark: The Nation's Unhealthiest City, 1832–1895*, Galishoff (1988) noted high death rates in Newark, and the South (with a large black population having death rates greater than those for whites).

Rates for black women 15–44 years old by MSA
The MSAs and PMSAs with the lowest and highest age-standardized death rates (ages 15–44 years) for black women are shown in Table 5-9; mortality data for all 50 MSAs and PMSAs are shown in Appendix Table A-9. Death rates were lower for women than for men for each race, and the lowest rates for black women (and lowest black/white ratios of rates) were for Anaheim–Santa Ana and San Jose. While the age-standardized death rates for black women were based on small numbers of deaths in Anaheim and San Jose, approximate upper 95% confidence limits were also low (i.e., <120 per 100,000 per year; data not shown). Noteworthy are the high age-standardized death rates for black women (Table 5-10) in several large MSAs in the Northeast and Midwest (as found for males). Rates of about 200 per 100,000 per year or greater were found for Baltimore, Chicago, Detroit, New York, and Newark. The highest black death rate and the highest black/white ratio of rates were for Newark (as found for men). Statistically, these high rates were quite reliable; standard errors for the age-standardized rates were relatively small because of the large numbers of deaths involved.

Rates in California MSAs
The larger California MSAs and PMSAs are useful in analyses of the association between segregation index and mortality rates because of the relatively wide range of black–white segregation indexes in the same state, as discussed earlier with regard to infant mortality rates.

Table 5-10. Black/white ratios of mortality rates for young adult females and age-standardized mortality rates (ages 15–44 years) in selected MSAs and PMSAs, 1990–1991*

MSA	Black/white ratios of age-specific rates			Age-standardized rates (ASRs)			Segregation index	Black poverty (percent)
	15–24	25–34	35–44	Black	White	Ratio		
LOWEST BLACK ASRs (<100)								
Anaheim	0.57	0.97	0.97	66.9	75.3	0.89	43	10
San Jose	0.59	1.14	1.42	74.7	62.7	1.19	45	13
HIGHEST BLACK ASRs (>200)								
Baltimore	1.77	2.96	3.28	201.6	69.3	2.91	75	23
Chicago	2.07	3.26	3.00	211.3	73.1	2.89	87	30
Fort Lauderdale	1.40	3.09	2.60	231.1	91.0	2.54	73	27
Miami	2.05	3.45	3.18	253.9	82.4	3.08	75	30
New York, NY	1.31	1.79	2.05	247.2	133.7	1.85	78	25
Newark	2.96	5.19	5.13	344.7	71.6	4.81	83	20

*For data on all 50 MSAs and PMSAs, see Appendix Tables. Age-standardized rates are per 100,000 per year.

Using numbers of deaths for males in 1987–1989 (from *Vital Statistics of the United States*) and the estimated black and white male populations (15–24 to 35–44 years old) of each MSA and PMSA for 1987–1989, age-specific rates (15–24 to 35–44 years) were standardized by the "direct" method, with the distribution of the 1980 U.S. population from age 15–24 to 35–44 as the "standard" population.

The black/white ratio of the age-standardized death rates in California MSAs and PMSAs (Table 5-11) tended to increase with rising level of black–white segregation. The black/white ratio of poverty rates in these seven MSAs and PMSAs also tended to increase as the segregation index increased. However, while Los Angeles had the highest black/white mortality ratio and the highest segregation index, it did not have the highest black/white poverty rate ratio. Except for Anaheim–Santa Ana and San Jose, poverty rates for blacks in all other MSAs and PMSAs were within a narrow range (20–24%), but mortality rates for blacks varied considerably and tended to increase with increasing level of segregation. Again, the low black/white ratios of age-standardized deaths rates in several MSAs are noteworthy. Numbers of deaths for black females in these MSAs were too small for meaningful analyses.

The clearest separation in the black/white ratio of mortality rates was between the five MSAs with lower segregation indexes and the two with the highest indexes (Los Angeles and San Francisco–Oakland or Oakland), except that Sacramento had a relatively high ratio (Table 5-11). The low black/white ratio of death rates for the Anaheim–Santa Ana MSA in 1990–1991 is especially noteworthy. This was due to an age-adjusted death rate for blacks that was lower than that for all other MSAs (Appendix Table A-8), with the exception of Riverside. The low death rate for whites in the Riverside MSA (relative to

Table 5-11. California MSAs: black/white ratios of mortality rates for males 15–44 years old (age-standardized rate) by time period

MSA*	Segregation index (1980)	Black/white death rate (1982–1986)	Black/white death rate (1987–1989)	Segregation index (1990)	Black poverty (1990)	Black/white death rate (1990–1991)
Anaheim	47	1.52	1.20	43	9.7	0.80
San Jose	48	1.14	1.32	45	12.7	1.28
Riverside	58	1.23	1.02	49	20.4	1.30
Sacramento	60	1.78	1.52	58	24.0	1.57
San Diego	63	1.34	1.36	59	21.3	1.28
San Francisco–Oakland	(68)	1.74	1.65	65	—	—
(Oakland)	75	—	—	69	21.1	1.60
Los Angeles	80	1.61	1.68	71	21.2	1.57

*Titles of MSAs have been abbreviated (see Appendix).

whites in the Anaheim MSA) resulted in a higher black/white ratio of age-adjusted death rates than for Anaheim (Appendix Table A-8).

Segregation and Poverty as Predictors: Older Adults (45–64 Years Old)

A consistent finding for decades has been that black–white differences in mortality rates (beyond infancy) are highest for young adults and that the black/white ratio declines after middle age (Chapter 4). The next analyses involved age-specific death rates for ages 45–54 and 55–64 for black and white men in the 50 MSAs; these rates are listed in Appendix Table A-10.

For black men, the association between black mortality rate and segregation index was statistically significant for ages 45–54 but not for ages 55–64, although the association was positive for both age groups (Appendix Table A-11). The black poverty rate was positively associated with the black mortality rate for both age groups, but the regression coefficients did not reach the conventional level (i.e., 0.05) of "statistical significance."

For black women, segregation was a significant predictor of death rates in both 45–54 and 55–64 year olds, while the black poverty rate was a stronger predictor in 55–64 olds (Appendix Table A-11). Mortality rates are listed in Appendix Table A-12.

With regard to the black/white ratio of death rates, the segregation index was not a significant predictor for men (Appendix Table A-11). This reflected the stronger associations between white poverty rate and white death rates than between black poverty rates and black death rates. Highly segregated MSAs in the East and Midwest tended to have very high black/white ratios of poverty rates; examples are Chicago, Detroit, Milwaukee, Minneapolis, Newark, New York, Philadelphia, St. Louis, and Washington, DC. These MSAs also had relatively high black/white ratios of death rates (Appendix Table A-10). Noteworthy was the importance of the black/white ratio of poverty rates as a predictor of the black/white ratio of mortality rates in both the 45–54- and 55–64-year-old age groups of men, while for women the association was weaker (Appendix Table A-11).

Among women 55–64 years old, the segregation index (and not the black/white poverty ratio) was a statistically significant predictor of the black/white ratio of death rates (Appendix Table A-11). Black/white ratios of death rates were low in certain MSAs in the west for ages 55–64, and some of these ratios were lower than those for ages 45–54 (Appendix Table A-12).

Quality of Housing and Neighborhood as Predictors

The next analyses focused on males aged 15–44 years because of the stronger associations between segregation and black mortality rates in this age group (vs. older ages) and the greater statistical reliability of these age-standardized death rates for men than women.

The association between level of segregation and black mortality rates could represent the effects of more proximal causal variables related to quality of life. Total homicide (i.e., murder and non-negligent manslaughter) rates for all races combined by MSA were obtained from *Uniform Crime Reports 1990*, published by the Federal Bureau of Investigation (1991). Data for most large MSAs, with a few exceptions, are included in these annual reports; thus, data were available for 46 of the 50 MSAs used in the previous analyses. The total homicide rate was a statistically significant predictor of the black and white death rates (ages 15–44 years, age-standardized). The segregation index was still a significant predictor of the age-standardized death rate for blacks, even when the total homicide rate was included in the model (Appendix Table A-13). In contrast to the findings for black men, the mortality rate for white men showed a slight negative correlation with the segregation index and a significant positive correlation with the white poverty rate by MSA.

The rate of violent crimes in 1990 by MSA was also used in regression models, but was not found to be an important predictor of variation in death rates for black men 15–44 years old or 45–54 to 55–64 years old. Data on both total homicide rate and quality of housing by race were available for 33 MSAs (listed in Appendix Table A-14). For both housing and neighborhood quality, the proportion of black households receiving a low or poor rating (1–4 on a scale of 10) were calculated (i.e., as described earlier for infant mortality). The segregation index was positively correlated with the proportion of black households with low ratings on quality of neighborhood and quality of household (Appendix Table A-15), as expected from the effects of black–white segregation on the quality of life for blacks in many urban areas (Chapter 3).

Multiple linear regression was used to predict the age-standardized death rate (ages 15–44 years) for black men in 1990–1991. The segregation index and the total homicide rate (all races, 1990) for the entire MSA were important predictors of the black mortality rate (Appendix Table A-16). The proportion of black householders that provided a rating for the neighborhood quality that was low (i.e., 1–4 on a 10-point scale, as described earlier) was not a statistically significant predictor. The statistical significance of segregation index even after the total homicide rate was included suggests a possible association between segregation and causes of death other than homicide. However, the homicide rate was the total rate for the entire MSA, and not for blacks alone. Other variables, not included in the model shown, were the black poverty rate, the proportion of black household units with 1.01 + persons per room (see Kitagawa and Hauser, 1973), and the proportion of housing units rated as low quality (1–4 on a 10-point scale). These variables made little contribution to the prediction of the black mortality rate when the segregation index was included in the model. While the association between black mortality rates and segregation could operate through these variables (Chapter 6), they have no significant effect on black mortality rates (males aged 15–44 years) independent of the effect of the segregation index.

Selected Causes of Death in 50 MSAs

Because the number of deaths from specific causes by MSA were not available for blacks and whites separately, analyses were limited to age-adjusted death rates (in 1990) for both sexes and all races combined using the same 50 MSAs involved in analyses of mortality in young adult males just described. Numbers of deaths for selected groups of causes were obtained from published national reports (*Vital Statistics of the United States*, U.S. Department of Health and Human Services, 1982–1990a), and population data are from the 1990 Census. The causes selected showed larger black–white differences in mortality rates in 1990, especially for young and middle-aged adults (see Table 4-1, and Chapter 4), including cardiovascular diseases (International Classification of Diseases [ICD], codes 390–448), nephritis and kidney diseases (ICD 580–589), and "homicides/legal interventions" (ICD E960–E968).

Differences in the age distribution of the population at risk across MSAs were taken into account by age standardization using the "indirect" method. Adjustment for differences in the ratios of males to females by MSA was not possible. The proportion of the total population of each MSA that was black and the segregation index in 1990 (Farley and Frey, 1994b) were included in all models (Appendix Table A-17), along with the black/white ratio of poverty rates (1990 Census) for each MSA. Not shown was the number of physicians (in 1988) per 100,000 population for each MSA, because this was a poor independent predictor of death rates. Use of the standardized mortality ratios (SMRs) by MSA rather than the age-standardized rates by MSA facilitates comparisons across MSAs. The SMRs were calculated as the ratio of the observed number of deaths from the specific cause in each MSA to the number expected on the basis of age-specific death rates for the specific cause of death in the entire United States in 1990.

Noteworthy were the low SMRs for certain MSAs in California (including Anaheim–Santa Ana). SMRs for cardiovascular diseases showed limited variability, while variation in SMRs for homicides was striking (Table 5-12).

The segregation index was a statistically significant predictor of the age-

Table 5-12. Standardized mortality ratios (SMRs) for all races combined
for selected causes in 50 MSAs in 1990

MSA*	Segregation index (1990)	Percent black	SMRs		
			Cardiovascular	Nephritis	Homicide
Anaheim	43	2	0.87	0.47	0.71
Atlanta	73	26	0.98	1.21	1.32
Baltimore	75	26	1.02	1.60	1.54
Baton Rouge	73	30	1.09	1.71	1.40
Birmingham	79	27	1.01	1.43	2.01
Boston	70	6	1.18	1.69	0.73
Buffalo	84	11	1.13	0.93	0.50
Charleston	58	30	1.07	1.26	0.87
Charlotte	65	20	1.04	1.00	1.40
Chicago	87	22	1.05	1.44	1.69
Cincinnati	80	13	1.02	1.12	0.56
Cleveland	86	19	1.05	1.18	1.15
Columbus	71	12	1.01	1.12	0.55
Dallas	66	16	1.01	0.53	1.93
Denver	66	6	0.81	0.59	0.63
Detroit	89	22	1.10	1.06	1.87
Fort Lauderdale	73	15	0.91	0.81	1.13
Greensboro	68	19	0.99	0.88	0.89
Houston	69	19	1.02	0.89	2.10
Indianapolis	80	14	0.99	1.51	0.76
Jackson, MS	75	42	1.09	1.19	1.69
Jacksonville	65	20	1.04	0.80	2.21
Kansas City	76	13	0.95	1.08	1.16
Los Angeles	71	11	1.04	0.70	2.07
Memphis	76	41	1.18	1.23	2.40
Miami	75	21	0.93	0.82	2.23

(continued)

adjusted death rate for cardiovascular diseases and approached statistical significance for nephritis and kidney diseases (Appendix Table A-17). For homicides, the poverty rate and proportion black were statistically significant predictors, but the segregation index did not reach statistical significance. The homicide rate was high in several southern MSAs (and highest in New Orleans) not
characterized by high segregation indexes (Table 5-12).

Future studies should consider age-specific and age-adjusted rates for blacks
and whites separately, although small numbers of deaths by cause for blacks
would necessitate combining data for several years.

Conclusion

In comparison with the findings for infant mortality, the results for mortality in
young adults (ages 15–44 years) were more consistent over time. A statistically
significant association between degree of black–white segregation and black
mortality rates (at least for males), apparently independent of social class vari-

Table 5-12. (Continued)

MSA*	Segregation index (1990)	Percent black	SMRs		
			Cardiovascular	Nephritis	Homicide
Milwaukee	84	14	0.98	0.97	1.14
Minneapolis	65	4	0.80	0.85	0.40
Nashville	66	15	1.08	0.98	0.89
Nassau and Suffolk Counties, NY	79	7	1.03	0.90	0.40
New Orleans	74	35	1.10	1.54	3.18
New York, NY	78	26	1.09	1.05	2.65
Newark	83	23	0.96	1.31	1.06
Norfolk	57	29	1.09	1.10	1.15
Oakland	69	15	0.93	0.93	1.27
Philadelphia	82	19	0.99	1.11	1.35
Phoenix	51	3	0.83	0.96	0.90
Pittsburgh	75	8	1.06	1.47	0.47
Portland	68	3	0.92	0.52	0.42
Raleigh	57	25	0.93	0.82	0.88
Richmond, VA	64	29	1.02	1.12	1.85
Riverside	49	7	1.01	0.49	1.37
Sacramento	58	7	0.89	0.93	0.67
St Louis	81	17	1.05	0.98	1.41
San Antonio	57	7	0.87	0.73	1.77
San Diego	59	6	0.85	0.60	0.84
San Jose	45	4	0.81	0.78	0.41
Seattle	60	4	0.84	0.42	0.50
Tampa	74	9	0.90	0.38	0.97
Washington, DC	68	27	0.86	1.17	1.66

*Titles of MSAs/PMSAs have been abbreviated (see Appendix).

ables (as measured in ecologic studies), was found for 1990–1991, as reported previously for 1982–1986. Statistical analyses (using multiple linear regression) showed that the segregation index by MSA was a predictor of black mortality rates for ages 15–44 years, while the black poverty rate was not a predictor.

A number of MSAs in the western part of the country continued to have relatively low death rates for young adult black males, and black/white ratios of death rates were also low (although rarely less than 1.00). Such low black/white ratios of death rates are remarkable in view of the considerable black–white differences in poverty rates and the absolute levels of black–white segregation by MSA. In contrast, several large, hypersegregated MSAs in the Northeast and Midwest had high black mortality rates.

The limitations of ecologic studies must be recognized. The analyses in this chapter are intended to provide further impetus for detailed studies that measure among individuals such variables as social class, segregation, and discrimination. In the emerging study of the epidemiology of American apartheid, the ecologic analyses described in this chapter also may stimulate interesting speculation regarding possible explanations, as well as suggest leads for future studies (Chapter 6).

6

Interpretations
and Research Needs

This discussion of the interpretation of the findings in Chapter 5 starts with problems inherent in the use of ecologic studies, along with various "errors of measurement" (MacMahon and Pugh, 1970). A consideration of potential explanations involving the concentration or neighborhood effects of segregation follows. Because the ecologic studies presented in this book serve mainly to generate hypotheses, the discussion is speculative. It involves mainly a review of the literature on the effects of discrimination in such areas as medical (health) care, quality of life issues for blacks (especially in inner cities), exposures to stresses, and certain psychosocial and physiologic responses to stress. This review deals with the epidemiology of discrimination and racism. It is intended to stimulate further studies of the association between segregation and the health of blacks. The final discussion concerns the need for further ecologic studies, with more detailed data than were available for Chapter 5, along with nonecologic (or "analytic") epidemiologic studies that obtain information on individuals.

The ecologic analyses of geographic variation in death rates in Chapter 5 also raised issues that go beyond the issue of the association between mortality and segregation or discrimination and racism. This is especially true for time trends in black infant mortality rates in different regions of the country, which are not explained by trends in segregation. Hypotheses involving temporal and regional changes in health care delivery, albeit speculative, are discussed in this chapter.

Limitations of Ecologic Studies

Biases

Issues of biases in ecologic studies have been considered mainly with regard to multiple linear regression models (Greenland and Robins, 1994a,b) such as those used in Chapter 5. A major problem concerns the inability to control **97** adequately for other factors, referred to as "covariates," that are potential "confounders." Confounders are factors that produce bias in epidemiologic studies, making it appear that an "exposure" of interest (that is, segregation) is involved in the causal chain leading to mortality among blacks. The prevalence rate of poverty or low income among blacks by MSA is a potential confounder, because it is associated both with the level of segregation and the black mortality rate by MSA. Many large, "older" MSAs in the East and Midwest have high black poverty rates as well as high levels of segregation and high death rates for blacks.

The arrows in Figure 6-1 indicate causal pathways or potential pathways. The correlation between black poverty rate and black–white residential segregation by MSA is indicated in Figure 6-1 by the line between "black poverty" and "segregation," as mentioned in Chapter 1 (Fig. 1-1). "Multicolinearity" refers to correlations between independent variables ("predictors" of mortality) that are so strong as to invalidate analyses using multiple regression. However, the correlation coefficients between segregation index and black poverty rate, in the analyses involving varying numbers of MSAs (Chapter 5), were not high enough to present a major obstacle. Also, within some groups of MSAs with similar black poverty rates, hypersegregated MSAs had high black mortality rates, as shown for MSAs in California (Chapter 5).

Ecologic studies usually lack detailed data on covariates (potential confounders) such as the distribution of income for blacks according to age and sex. Black poverty rates for entire MSAs and PMSAs were used in Chapter 5. The overall *distribution* of income among all residents or households, which is related to mortality (Chapter 4), also could differ among MSAs, even among those with similar black poverty rates. This "distribution" issue is distinct from that of the *geographic* distribution of poverty (or low income), which is affected by segregation (Chapter 3).

Statistical "control" for the covariate (income or social class) may be inadequate. Ecologic studies often use county-level summaries (or, in our analyses, the multi-county MSA unit) such as median household or family income, which are "not sufficient to create internally homogeneous strata" (Greenland and Robins, 1994b). Such summary statistics can be especially inadequate when associations are nonlinear or when interactions between variables are involved.

However, the regression analyses in Chapter 5 also included, in addition to black poverty rates by MSA, data on segments of the distribution of race-specific household income for each MSA. Analyses that used the proportions of

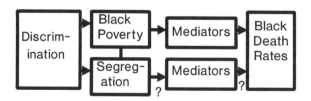

Figure 6-1. Black poverty (low income) as a potential confounder in the association between segregation and black mortality.

blacks and whites in the lowest income levels in each MSA produced results from regression models that were similar to those obtained by using "group" (population) data on total poverty rates for black and white persons by MSA.

Examination of the distribution of incomes for black households in selected MSAs (Table 6-1) in 1989, from the 1990 Census, shows that five of the seven large MSAs in California used in the analyses in Chapter 5 not only had similar black poverty rates and median incomes for black households but also had similar proportions of black households with low incomes (i.e., <$5,000, $5,000–$9,999, and $10,000–$14,999). The proportions of black persons with an income that was less than 50% of the federal poverty level were also similar in these five MSAs. Nevertheless, the age-standardized death rate for black males 15–44 years in 1990–1991 (as presented also in Chapter 5) increased with increasing level of black–white segregation index among these MSAs (Table 6-1). For the two other California MSAs used in Chapter 5 (i.e., Anaheim–Santa Ana and San Jose), both the black income levels and segregation indexes were low, along with the death rates for young adult black men.

Data for two MSAs in the Northeast with black poverty rates roughly similar to those for the five California MSAs are also shown for comparison (Table 6-1). While the distributions were similar in most respects, the proportion of black households with very low incomes (less than $5,000) was higher in both New York City and Newark than in the California MSAs (Fig. 6-2). This could help to explain the high death rates for black men (aged 15–44 years) in these two northeastern MSAs than in the California MSAs (see also Appendix tables).

Another problem could not be addressed. Mortality rates are often age stan-

Table 6-1. Distribution (percent of households) of income (in 1989) of black households, and other income measures, in selected MSAs*

	California MSAs					Northeast MSAs	
	Los Angeles	Oakland	Sacramento	San Diego	Riverside	Newark	New York
Households (1000s)	350	111	34	50	54	140	758
Income							
<$5,000	8%	8%	7%	6%	6%	10%	13%
$5,000–$9,999	14%	15%	15%	12%	11%	11%	12%
$10,000–$14,999	9%	10%	11%	11%	10%	7%	8%
Median ($)	25,827	24,840	23,731	25,125	28,474	27,995	24,278
Poverty							
<50%	9%	9%	9%	8%	8%	11%	14%
<100%	21%	21%	24%	21%	20%	20%	25%
<125%	27%	27%	32%	28%	27%	24%	30%
Segregation index	71	69	58	59	49	83	78
Death rate (ages 15–44 years)	567	550	370	282	189	772	747

*Death rate is age standardized (see Chapter 5). Poverty rates are for all black persons in each MSA for whom poverty was determined, as reported by the 1990 Census. Poverty of "<50%" refers to incomes less than half of the federal poverty level (Chapter 3).

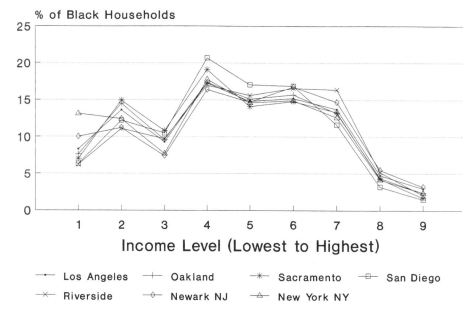

Figure 6-2. Distribution of black household income (1989) for five MSAs in California and two in the Northeast; 1 = less than \$5,000; 2 = \$5,000–\$9,999; 3 = \$10,000–\$14,999; 4 = \$15,000–\$24,999; 5 = \$25,000–\$34,999; 6 = \$35,000–\$49,999; 7 = \$50,000–\$74,999; 8 = \$75,000–\$99,999; 9 = \$100,000 or more.

dardized, thus taking into account differences in the distribution of age across MSAs. However, such ecologic "exposure" variables as segregation index and poverty rate (or income distributions) are usually not age standardized (Greenland and Robins, 1994a,b). While some analyses in Chapter 5 involved use of age-specific death rates, data for corresponding age strata (and by gender) were not available for segregation and social class indicators.

Other Methodologic Problems and Issues

The problem of migration in ecologic studies was not considered by Greenland and Robins (1994a,b) or in the analyses in Chapter 5. Long "latency" periods, or time intervals between initiation of exposures to causal factors and the onset of disease, are involved in chronic diseases. Exposures initiated during childhood and early adult life may be crucial. Social class during childhood, in addition to current or recent social class, may be related to mortality in later life (Peck, 1994). Only intensive studies, analytic rather than ecologic in design, can address the issue of inadequate adjustment for social class.

Residential mobility would affect the ability of ecologic studies to detect associations between current levels of "exposure" and death rates. However, the small declines in segregation in many large MSAs indicate that black mobility is limited (Chapter 2). Some migration of blacks to smaller MSAs with small proportions of blacks and lower segregation has occurred, and there could be residual health effects of previous experiences in ghettos. However, chronic "exposures" to certain environmental factors and persistently poor access to (and quality of) medical care would have effects on current death rates for blacks; thus, time of migration to the geographic area under study would have less impact on the interpretation of death rates by area.

Another issue involves the restricted range of segregation found among the MSAs and PMSAs studied. Segregation index is a continuous "exposure" variable, with a theoretical range of 0–100, but there are very few MSAs with even medium levels of black–white segregation (Chapter 2). This also holds for black poverty rates by MSA. Different findings might be obtained if there were MSAs with lower levels of segregation and/or black poverty, depending on the nature of the associations. This has implications for the potential impact on health of interventions to reduce black poverty rates and black–white segregation. By way of possible analogy, international studies of mortality rates in relation to specific dietary factors (such as dietary fat intake) involve greater variation in this "exposure" variable than studies within a single country (such as the United States). This has implications for conclusions about the etiologic role of dietary fat in various chronic diseases and the potential benefits of large changes in diet.

The regression equations (as shown in Chapter 5) could be used to "predict" mortality rates for blacks residing in MSAs with lower segregation levels than those actually included in the analyses, but the results would be of only theoretical interest in the absence of MSAs with lower levels of segregation than those involved in Chapter 5. Future studies could combine many smaller MSAs with low levels of segregation that were not included in Chapter 5. Problems would include small numbers of annual deaths and potential regional (geographic) factors affecting mortality among MSAs in widely scattered areas.

Some of the death rates for blacks by MSA (Chapter 5) involved small black populations and small numbers of deaths among blacks (by gender) for a given year or even several years combined. Caution was urged in the interpretation of black death rates for individual MSAs. Because MSAs with the lowest segregation tend to have small populations (especially of blacks), the statistical precision of the death rates for blacks in these small MSAs is lower than that for larger MSAs. However, groups of MSAs defined by level of segregation were included in some analyses that attempted to discern a pattern related to mortality rates. The comparability of infant death rates over time was affected by changes in the definition of "black" infant mortality rates, but the effect was probably small. Finally, the segregation indexes used in the regression analyses (Chapter 5) were for "Anglos" (non-Hispanic whites) and blacks, while death rates were for all whites and blacks. In geographic areas with large Hispanic populations, especially in parts of California and the Southwest, the populations for which segregation indexes were measured may not correspond well with the populations for which white death rates were estimated. Overall death rates for all ages and all causes of death combined for "Hispanics," an extremely diverse racial-ethnic group (Chapter 2), tend to be lower than those for non-Hispanic whites (Polednak, 1995; Sorlie et al., 1993).

Another problem concerns errors in the data rather than issues of statistical uncertainty or definitions of groups. Census undercounts, especially for young adult black men (Chapter 4), may vary in magnitude among MSAs, resulting in differential overestimation of death rates for black men in these age groups. However, the magnitude of variation in these death rates across MSAs was probably too great (Chapter 5) for such errors to be a major explanation. Also, associations between segregation and black mortality rates by MSA were found for older age groups among men (45–54 year olds) and for black women (Chapter 5).

Conceptual Framework: Further Details

Segregation itself is not a direct "cause" of mortality, but rather a marker for other factors that may be "mediators" between segregation and mortality in blacks (Figs. 6-1 and 6-3). There are many potential mediators or more direct causal factors in the causal chain from segregation to mortality among blacks. These factors could not be considered in the analyses in Chapter 5 because of the lack of data on blacks and whites by MSA, as discussed in the next section. Any effects of segregation could occur independent of social class. That is, both poor and nonpoor blacks could be adversely affected by living in highly segregated areas. However, segregation could interact with social class in complex ways to affect the health of urban blacks that could not be adequately addressed in Chapter 5.

Concentration or neighborhood effects (Chapter 3) relate to the epidemiology of American apartheid. Examples are high rates of unwed mothers per 1,000 live births, poor access to and quality of medical care, crime and illicit drug use, violence, and the physical deterioration of neighborhoods. The possible roles of variation in levels of black community empowerment, crowding, and exposure to toxic agents in the general (ambient) and occupational environment

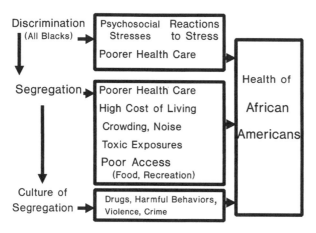

Figure 6-3. Conceptual framework, expanded from Figure 1-1.

(Fig. 6-3) are discussed as "neighborhood" factors for urban blacks. Again, the relationship between these factors and degree of segregation has not been studied.

The high cost of living in ghettos (Fig. 6-3) is another issue, as noted for predominantly nonwhite New York City areas (Yankauer, 1950). Housing costs or gross rent as a percentage of household income reportedly increased as much in one urban ghetto area (East Harlem), despite the higher poverty rate (and hence, lower ability to pay), as in other areas of New York City in the 1980s (Freidenberg, 1995). Differences in cost of living for blacks in MSAs that differ in segregation could modify the impact of income and thereby affect variation in black mortality rates by MSA. Apparently, data on cost of living are not available for blacks and whites in specific metropolitan areas (Jencks, 1993). Therefore, adjustment for such variations in analyses of mortality by MSA is not possible.

Some pathways in Figure 6-3 are not dependent on segregation and are part of the broader area of the epidemiology of discrimination and racism. Quality of medical care may be poorer for blacks than whites (due to discrimination), independent of social class and irrespective of the level of segregation in the neighborhood. Psychosocial stresses, and reactions to these stresses, may be important for all blacks regardless of where they live. Responses to experiences with discrimination and racism (as stressors) may contribute to health problems in blacks regardless of the level of segregation in current or past residential areas. In spite of "class differences" (and, it might be added, place of residence), all blacks are "the targets, to greater or lesser degrees, of some form of racist assault" (hooks, 1995). Although hooks speculated that less-privileged blacks may be more likely to experience racism, there are apparently few objective studies. Small-scale studies suggest that discrimination is experienced by middle-class and professional blacks, but the effects may be reduced among higher social classes due to better resources (Feagin, 1991), as discussed later. Experiences with discrimination and responses to these experiences apparently have not been studied among blacks (of different social classes) living in areas that differ in level of segregation. The following discussion is largely restricted to the epidemiology of discrimination and racism and the limited evidence for interactions with social class with regard to hypertension.

Infant Mortality: Interpretations

In the ecologic analyses in Chapter 5, the black/white ratio of poverty rates by MSA was a significant predictor of the black/white ratio of infant mortality rates by MSA. However, the amount of variation accounted for was small, especially by around 1990. The literature has shown that control for single factors related to social class, such as maternal or parental education, is not sufficient to account for black–white differences in adverse pregnancy outcomes. One study of black college-educated parents (Hogue and Hargreaves, 1993; Schoendorf et al., 1992) is often cited to show the persistence of higher rates of low birth weight (a major risk factor for infant mortality) in blacks than in whites. Therefore, black–white social class differences as measured in a limited fashion and within a single generation do not explain all of the black–white differences in the frequency of adverse pregnancy outcomes.

Black poverty rate by MSA was not a predictor of variation in black infant mortality among 92 MSAs in 1989–1991 in regression models that included the segregation index. The correlation of black infant mortality was stronger with the segregation index than with the black poverty rate by MSA. However, the range of black poverty rates was limited. Only 4 of 92 MSAs analyzed for 1989–1991, and only 6 of the 103 MSAs used in the analyses of 1991 infant mortality rates had a black poverty rate of less than 20% in the 1990 Census. In addition, numerous researchers have pointed out the possibility that intergenerational factors might affect the offspring of black mothers. This is especially relevant to blacks because, although the middle class has grown in recent decades, past generations were poorer. Black mothers currently under study could be affected by factors related to the social class of their own mothers (e.g., body size and nutritional factors). An intergenerational study is in progress at Meharry Medical College (Nashville, TN) examining birth weights of black and white infants across several generations, including groups with sustained high socioeconomic status (Foster et al., 1993).

However, the considerable variation in black infant mortality rates by MSA (Fig. 4-2) was largely unexplained in the analyses in Chapter 5. While the segregation index (rather than the black poverty rate) was a predictor of black infant mortality rates in 1989–1991, little of the variation in rates was "explained" by the model. This reflects the paucity of variables included in the model due to lack of available information by MSA.

Data on specific variables that have been associated with adverse pregnancy outcomes in black women were not available by MSA. In epidemiologic studies of selected groups, statistical control for multiple risk factors that differed in prevalence between black and white mothers removed most (if not all) black–white differences in prematurity and/or low birth weight (Shiono et al., 1986; Lieberman et al., 1987; Wise and Pursley, 1992; Rawlings et al., 1995). Examples of the risk factors analyzed in these studies are maternal age (especially teenage motherhood), aspects of timing and quality of prenatal care, marital status (unmarried vs. married), and certain medical risk factors. Actual "control" (i.e., amelioration) of these risk factors in real black populations remains a sociopolitical, medical, and public health challenge in order to reduce black–white disparities in infant mortality. Nutritional factors are also important, as shown by studies of birth defects (one cause of infant death) and low birth weight.

While the importance of segregation as a predictor of black infant mortality rates declined over time during the 1980s, high black infant mortality rates persisted over time in certain hypersegregated MSAs. Concentration or neighborhood effects are relevant to many of these variables, including the "rate" of unwed mothers (Chapter 5). Some of these factors may "mediate" the effect of living in hypersegregated areas on black infant mortality rates. The ultimate causes of higher rates of unwed mothers (among women of childbearing age and among all live births) in blacks, especially in inner cities, may be related to neighborhood effects and the culture of segregation (Chapter 3). Illicit drug use in young adults, for example, is affected by neighborhood of residence (Chapter 3) and is associated with a variety of pregnancy complications and adverse pregnancy outcomes (Robins and Mills, 1993), although it is only a minor factor in explaining black infant mortality.

Various factors (including medical care, stress, and nutrition) that might be related to discrimination and racism are discussed below. The potential role of segregation cannot be delineated. Also, the discussion is not limited to the potential role of discrimination and racism or segregation.

Medical Care

The distinction between neonatal and postneonatal death rates (Chapter 5) is important in the interpretation of variation in overall infant death rates because different factors have been shown to influence neonatal and postneonatal death rates. Prenatal and (especially) neonatal medical care is important in affecting neonatal death rates and time trends in these rates. Postnatal medical care and postnatal environmental quality, such as nutritional factors and exposure to infections, affect postneonatal mortality rates.

An intervention study in West Virginia demonstrates the potential importance of medical care in relation to postneonatal death rates. Infants at high risk for postneonatal death, due to maternal characteristics and medical history, were provided with a medical care intervention that included a schedule of postnatal physician visits and provision of home monitors for medical problems related to risk of sudden infant death syndrome and heart arrhythmias. The intervention was followed by a much larger reduction in the statewide postneonatal infant mortality rate than occurred in three similar (mainly rural) states over the same time period, suggesting that the intervention might have had an impact (Myerberg et al., 1995). The relevance of these findings to this discussion is that geographic variation in the quality of postnatal medical care for black infants, related to or independent of variation in social class of blacks, could influence geographic variation in postneonatal mortality rates for blacks. Similarly, temporal changes in such medical care could affect temporal changes in these mortality rates.

Adverse effects of discrimination and racism and segregation
The findings of Yankauer's study in New York City (1950) showing a slightly greater association between percentage of nonwhites in the population and postneonatal rather than neonatal infant mortality rates (Chapter 5 and Table 5-1) are intriguing. Unfortunately, neonatal and postneonatal death rates are not published by MSA, and special studies in specific MSAs and PMSAs are needed.

With regard to the epidemiology of discrimination and racism, an example involving a medical procedure, cesarean delivery, that may be unnecessary in some women may be illustrative. After controlling for various personal and hospital characteristics among hospital discharges for live births in California, black women were 24% more likely than white women to undergo caesarean delivery, except among low-birth-weight and county-hospital births (Braveman et al., 1995). The findings could reflect differences in the racial attitudes of providers and "unconscious differences in how options are presented," as well as differences in actual reactions or preferences among patients and the availability of social support.

More research is needed in this area, as also shown by the results of a national study comparing the quality of medical advice for prenatal care given to black and white mothers (after adjusting for social class) (Kogan et al., 1994). Although discrimination could affect infant mortality independently of segregation (Figs. 1-1 and 6-2), studies are needed to determine if discrimination by providers varies across areas that differ in degree of black–white residential segregation.

Other hypotheses related to medical care
As noted earlier, analyses of time trends and geographic variations in death rates for infants may suggest hypotheses not necessarily related to segregation or discrimination and racism.

Black postneonatal mortality in both the Pacific (including California) and Mountain divisions increased slightly from 1984–1986 to 1989–1991 (reaching 7.3 and 7.6); changes for whites were small. An increase in black (but not white) infant mortality noted in parts of California during the 1980s was interpreted in terms of changes (after around 1985) in state health policy, with increasing emphasis on privatization and client case management that was not community oriented (Gates-Williams et al., 1992). Again, this is a speculative conclusion that requires closer examination through in-depth studies of the health care delivery systems (for blacks) in specific MSAs.

Only the New England area (or division as defined by the Bureau of the Census) and three southern divisions (South Atlantic, East South Central, and West South Central) showed declines in black *postneonatal* death rates from 1984–1986 to 1989–1991 (National Center for Health Statistics, 1994). For Massachusetts blacks the decline from 1984–1986 to 1989–1991 was greater for the postneonatal (from 6.3 to 3.8 or [−40%]) than the neonatal (from 13.6 to 9.7 [−29%]) rate. The Boston metropolitan area showed a decline in black infant mortality rate between 1985 and 1992 (Chapter 5). It was hypothesized that a 50% decline for blacks in the City of Boston between 1990 and 1992 might be due (at least in part) to black community empowerment programs developed to reduce the high black infant mortality rate and to prepare for the 1991 federally funded Healthy Start Initiative (Plough and Olafson, 1994). This hypothesis requires further examination.

A negative association between "relative black political power" and black postneonatal mortality was found among 176 U.S. cities in 1981–1985 (LaVeist, 1992). Absolute black political power was defined as the percentage of blacks on the city council and relative black political power as the ratio of this percentage to the percentage in the voting age population for the years under study

(LaVeist, 1993). Black political power was *higher* in highly segregated cities. LaVeist (1993) speculated that in a highly segregated black community further increasing the level of political power could reduce some the adverse consequences of segregation that affect pregnancy outcome in blacks. The mechanisms through which political power might affect black infant (postneonatal) mortality rates are unknown, although effects on postnatal medical care (as well as quality of the environment) could be explored.

Psychosocial Stresses and "Neighborhood" Factors

Discrimination and/or segregation may be a proxy for the prevalence of multiple risk factors (including psychosocial stresses) relevant to adverse pregnancy outcome (Rowley and Tosteson, 1993; Edwards et al., 1994a,b).

A study in a highly segregated area may provide a model for other investigations and interventions. An intensive 5-year prospective study of a cohort of 443 urban African-American women 18–35 years old who attended prenatal clinics at Howard University Hospital (HUH) and the District of Columbia Department of Health Services was initiated in 1985; all pregnancies were delivered at HUH (Edwards et al., 1994a,b). The low-birth-weight rate achieved by the project (8.3%) was lower than that for black women seen at the same prenatal clinics but who were not part of the project (21.9%) and almost as low as that for private patients in the same area (6.3%). The HUH project involved prenatal visits, with social and psychological care, involving a "sense of caring" by clinic staff.

The possible roles of environmental stresses and racism experienced by blacks were emphasized, and it was hypothesized that the apparent effectiveness of the intervention was due in part to the psychosocial aspects of the care provided. Psychosocial variables were assessed by various instruments in the study, including a version of the Life Events Inventory and related scales designed to capture (albeit imperfectly) various stressful life experiences. Other instruments used in the HUH study evaluated self-image and social interactions. Evidence was marshalled in support of the hypothesis that self-attitudes may have been important. Racial identification scales for blacks were discussed in Chapter 2. Finally, improvements in compliance with WIC Program (Chapter 3) food and vitamin-mineral supplements also may have been important. However, in such multifaceted interventions it is difficult to "tease out" the components that were effective (and cost effective), and further studies are needed that emphasize particular components of the intervention at HUH.

Further studies are also needed to address the issue of whether the model devised by the Howard University intervention program can be applied to other settings. The study also suggests specific variables that should be examined in comparative and descriptive (nonintervention) studies across MSAs and PMSAs, such as detailed information on quality of postnatal care (including psychosocial support for pregnant women).

Clues to the causes of continued high black infant mortality rates in hypersegregated MSAs have been provided by in-depth studies of trends in low birth weight and infant mortality rates in New York City (Wallace and Wallace, 1990; Struening et al., 1990). After a period of destruction of housing and community institutions ("contagious urban decay") in the South Bronx, the temporal decline in the proportion of low-birth-weight births continued for predominantly white areas but not for predominantly black areas. The distribution of birth weights in blacks changed over time (with a higher maximum proportion of low weights) (Table 5-2). Also, a reversal of the trend of declining nonwhite infant death rates for all of New York City started to occur around the time the neighborhoods deteriorated.

Another concentration or neighborhood effect involves the use of illicit drugs, specifically cocaine (Chapter 3). Analysis of time trends in rates of low birth weight (a major factor in infant mortality) in New York City showed increases among blacks beginning in 1984, peaking in 1988, and then falling slightly. Because of the high prevalence of prenatal exposure to cocaine in such areas an Central Harlem and Flatbush (Brooklyn), the ecologic analyses suggested the hypothesis of an effect of trends in cocaine use on the trend in low birth weight (Joyce and Racine, 1993).

Research in other countries suggests that patterns of maternal social ties, rather than perceived exposure to stresses themselves, may mediate the effects of social class on infant health (Hagoel et al., 1995). Such variables as social ties and responses to stresses should be examined for black mothers residing in areas that differ in level of segregation. Detailed studies of infant mortality in specific hypersegregated MSAs, along with evidence from the 15 cities or intervention neighborhoods in the Healthy Start Initiative) (O'Campo et al., 1993), may provide an impetus for a sociopolitical commitment to expand interventions to accelerate the (slow) decline in the black infant mortality rate (Chapter 7). Baltimore and several other hypersegregated MSAs were chosen for the Healthy Start Initiative because of their high infant death rates.

In 1911–1916 in eight U.S. cities in the North and North Central regions, within groups defined by father's income, blacks had infant mortality rates only about 10% higher than those for native whites, and no black disadvantage was evident among infants of low-income mothers not employed outside the home (Ewbank, 1987). The rise in residential segregation in the North, after the migration of blacks to northern ghettos after World War I and World War II (Chapter 2), may have led to the emergence of factors that influenced black infant mortality independent of socioeconomic status (p. 83). This hypothesis requires further examination, although historical records may be difficult to obtain (especially for social class variables).

Quality of neighborhood for black households had a marginal impact on prediction of black infant death rates by MSA, independent of the segregation index (Chapter 5). However, these analyses are of limited value because of problems with the data available from the Census of Housing on quality of housing units occupied by black householders. In Chicago, as in many other areas, high black–white segregation means that blacks (regardless of income) tend to reside in census tracts with high poverty rates. The finding that even black infants with "adequate" prenatal care and full-term gestation had high neonatal death rates suggested a role for factors such as housing and nutrition, as well as various stresses and the quality of medical care in segregated (predominantly black) areas (Collins and David, 1992).

A few studies have shown an association between short interpregnancy interval and adverse pregnancy outcomes in black mothers (Rawlings et al., 1995), suggesting that this variable should be considered in analyzing geographic variation in black infant mortality rates. The high rates of birth to black teenage mothers in ghettos are noteworthy in this regard, although the explanation for such high rates is complex (Chapter 3).

Higher infant mortality rates for U.S. blacks than whites are due to both higher rates of low birth weight in blacks and higher black death rates within normal-birth-weight (but not within low-birth-weight) infants. Additional modeling studies are needed to evaluate the effect of segregation on infant mortality due to (and independent of) an association with low birth weight. A study showing high low-birth-weight rates in biracial infants of black mothers (mentioned in Chapter 2) has raised the possibility of adverse effects of stress, possibly due in part to discrimination and racism experienced by black mothers (Collins and David, 1993), and this hypothesis requires examination. Other studies suggest that intensive prenatal care, reduction in stress, and control of idiopathic premature labor may be required to reduce the black–white difference in low-birth-weight rates (Michielutte et al., 1994).

The extent of participation by black women in multiple public assistance programs (especially WIC and Medicaid), linked with reductions in infant mortality in some states (Rafferty, 1992), also should be considered when interpreting variation in black infant mortality rates by MSA. In Georgia, for example, high-risk women who were participants in WIC and Medicaid programs had lower infant mortality rates than nonparticipants, after adjusting for differences between the two groups in the frequency of the risk factors examined (i.e., teenage mothers, nonwhite rate, less than high school education, and inadequate prenatal care) (Rafferty, 1992) (Table 6-2). These risk factors are common among blacks in inner city areas. Geographic variation in black infant mortality rates could be influenced by variation in participation in (and in the effectiveness

Table 6-2. Odds ratios for infant mortality rates for infants of high-risk mothers who did and did not participate in public assistance programs in Georgia (1987)*

Program	Odds ratio	95% CI
WIC only	0.58	0.54–0.63
Medicaid only	0.64	0.49–0.85
Both	0.38	0.28–0.51

From Rafferty (1992).
* An odds ratio of 1.00 would indicate no difference in infant mortality rate between participants and nonparticipants.

of) such programs. Again, the relationship between these variables and degree of residential segregation have not been studied.

Conclusions

The specific environmental factors involved in the persistently high black infant mortality rates in hypersegregated MSAs have yet to be delineated, but there is no shortage of hypotheses to be explored. Segregation could be involved through its association with the concentration of high poverty rates for blacks. Mediators could include medical care factors, psychosocial stresses, the availability of social support and social ties, and other quality-of-life variables related to housing and nutritional factors (including poor access in ghettos to high-quality food at reasonable prices).

Disregarding the effects of segregation, studies are needed for the few instances where relatively low black infant death rates have been achieved, as in Boston in 1990 and 1991. In general, studies of changes in health service delivery and in black community empowerment offer promise for understanding time trends in black infant mortality rates. More important, such studies could provide information useful in planning interventions to improve black pregnancy outcomes.

Studies on psychosocial stresses in black mothers, and resources to deal with such stresses (including social support mechanisms), could identify more rapidly modifiable risk factors. Some modification of these risk factors could be achieved without addressing the underlying social and economic problems. Social and environmental problems in inner cities, such as those related to crime and illicit drug use, may not be easily modifiable, but one study (Edwards et al., 1994a,b) suggests that interventions at prenatal clinics may ameliorate the effects of adverse environments for black mothers and reduce rates of low-birth-weight infants (a major factor in infant mortality). Additional studies are needed on inner-city black women modeled after the apparently successful project at Howard University Hospital. Different combinations of interventions should be tested to identify specific components (e.g., social and psychological support by project staff, nutritional supplements, and stress reduction techniques) that were most effective (and cost effective).

A report from the Healthy Start Program in Baltimore (O'Campo et al., 1993) concluded that women in several areas of the city needed improved access to family planning services. The few studies conducted have suggested that adverse pregnancy outcomes in black women may be related to short intervals between births (mentioned earlier), which is due in part to neighborhood or concentration effects (Chapter 3). Thus, interventions aimed at child spacing could prove useful, but this requires further examination.

Adult Mortality: Interpretations

This section considers possible explanations for variations in death rates for black adults (and black/white ratios of rates) that might occur due to the concentration or neighborhood effects of segregation or to the culture of segregation and might interact with social class in complex ways. The specific relevance of segregation cannot be addressed. The discussion involves the more general topic of black–white differences in mortality that might be related to medical care and quality of life, after adjustment for social class, with implications for the epidemiology of discrimination and racism and the need for studies that consider degree of black–white residential segregation.

Medical Care

In 1896, E. Harris, a white professor at W.E.B. Du Bois's alma mater (Fisk University) remarked that "[S]ocial ostracism . . . and the discriminations which are made against the black man at least have no immediate bearing on his health, vitality, or longevity" (in "Social and Physical Condition of Negroes in Cities," 1896, quoted by Lewis, 1993, pp. 218–219). This statement was made in the first of the annual research publications of the Atlanta Conferences on "Negro problems" prior to Du Bois' stewardship starting with the conferences in 1897. Contrary to Harris' proclamation, access to medical care has always been a problem for black Americans. Numerous cases of denial of medical care at "white" hospitals (especially in the South) even for middle-class blacks, and even in critical emergency situations, during the mid-twentieth century contributed to the rise of "black" hospitals (Gamble, 1995).

Today, access to and quality of medical care may still differ for blacks and whites (American Medical Association, 1990) within each level of social class due to the effects of discrimination and racism. Whether such racism differs in extent for blacks living in areas that differ by level of segregation is apparently not known. However, populations at highest risk for medical problems (such as poor urban blacks) may have "limited contact with the health care system except in emergencies" (McCord and Freeman, 1990). The effects of poorer access to and poorer quality of medical care, along with poorer quality of life, on death rates for blacks in segregated areas requires further consideration.

In the long-term debate over the importance of quality of medical care in explaining declines in mortality rates, McKeown (1976) has emphasized the role of improvements in sanitation and hygiene or general amelioration of environmental conditions. Studies of overall mortality across countries with and without universal health insurance programs suggest that better access to health care may have limited impact on reducing disparities in morbidity and mortality by social class or income level (Adler et al., 1993; Najman, 1993). In reviews of "actual" causes of death in the United States, quantifying the impact of lack of access to primary care was problematic. One estimate was that about 7% of premature deaths and 15% of potential years of life lost before age 65 years are due to inadequate primary care (McGinnis and Foege, 1993). Thus, access to care for poor and minority persons should not be considered in isolation from other mechanisms involved in explaining disparities in health status by social class and race. This point has been noted with regard to the "perinatal paradox" (mentioned in Chapter 1).

While the importance of overall quality of life and environment must be emphasized, this does not preclude a role for access to (and quality of) care in explaining black–white differences in "preventable" deaths (Woolhander et al., 1989) and geographic variation in death rates for blacks.

Deaths from certain infectious and chronic diseases, especially among young adults, that can be largely prevented by proper diagnosis and treatment are "sentinel" events, indicative of failures of the health care system (Rutstein et al., 1976; Schwartz et al., 1990). Hospital admissions involving hypertension "emergencies" due to severe uncontrolled hypertension seen at emergency rooms in New York City were compared with hospital controls; black and Hispanic males predominated among the cases. Lack of a primary-care physician and health insurance, as well as a related pattern of receiving care at hospital emergency rooms rather than physicians' offices, were associated with noncompliance with treatment and the occurrence of hypertension emergencies in this case–control epidemiologic study (Shea et al., 1992a,b).

"Preventable" causes of death (including hypertension) were common among blacks in the District of Columbia, where the highest black–white disparities in death rates in 1980–1986 were from tuberculosis, certain other lung diseases, and hypertensive heart disease. This suggested that racial inequities in access to and quality of health care, in addition to "social conditions," were important (Schwartz et al., 1990).

In Chicago, asthma mortality rates increased continuously from 1968 to 1991 (by a total of 337% over the entire period) among African Americans 5–34 years old but remained constant among whites after 1976. A shift from hospital inpatients to non-inpatients (i.e., users of emergency departments and outpatient clinics) occurred among black asthma patients, suggesting an important role for changes in access to care (Targonski et al., 1994).

"Sentinel" events include deaths from "preventable" diseases at a relatively young age, such as diabetes and heart disease. Among hospitalized residents of New York State in 1983, more than 17,000 deaths and 336,000 instances of disease in a hospital discharge data base were regarded as possibly "avoidable." Higher rates of such deaths were found for blacks, along with Medicaid recipients and users of public (vs. private) hospitals (Carr et al., 1989). Significantly fewer deaths were prevented among hospitalized blacks than whites. For vascular complications of heart or brain associated with hypertensive disease, the black excess in age-adjusted case-fatality rates was 37%. Carr et al. (1989) emphasized the need for outreach and follow-up programs for patients with hypertension and other chronic diseases. Also mentioned were problems with accuracy of the data on race and ethnicity, as discussed in Chapter 2.

The common thread in all of these studies appears to be poorer primary care for blacks, especially in inner cities. Highly relevant to this issue, the estimated total number of African-American physicians (U.S. citizens) in 1991 was about 16,282, or lower than the 21,538 estimated in 1990 by the Bureau of the Census and a small proportion of the total of 562,350 U.S. physicians estimated for 1990 (King and Bendel, 1994). After rising for 7 years, the number of black applicants to U.S. medical schools declined between 1994 and 1995, although the significance of this short-term trend is unclear (Firshein, 1995). Most studies show that black (relative to white) physicians tend to see larger numbers of black and medically indigent patients, including uninsured and Medicaid patients (Moy and Bartman, 1995). With regard to ecologic studies in the epidemiology of American apartheid, data are needed on the proportion of blacks having a black physician in specific MSAs and PMSAs.

The specific causes of death that contributed to the association between segregation and total black mortality in young adults were not identified (Chapter 5). However, the black–white ratio of death rates for cardiovascular and cerebrovascular diseases in young adults is high (Table 4-1), and death rates from these diseases should be considered in future studies of the association between segregation and mortality in blacks. Studies of diagnostic and treatment services among adults hospitalized for heart disease have found that certain black–white disparities persist after adjustment for socioeconomic indicators by census tract of residence, as reviewed elsewhere (Ford and Cooper, 1995). Under-use by blacks, rather than unnecessary use of these procedures by whites, seems to be involved. As noted in Chapter 2, not all hospital discharge data bases include a "race" item; this should be a requirement for compliance with the 1964 Civil Rights Act (Title VI) (Watson, 1994).

In Veterans Administration (VA) hospitals, care is free and black–white socioeconomic differences among patients are smaller than in the general population, so that effects of social class differences should be largely eliminated. In a study of VA hospital patients, the number of major coronary procedures was lower for black than for white patients with acute myocardial infarction. However, 2-year survival rates did not differ (Peterson et al., 1994). While studies are needed on black–white differences in quality of life after hospitalization (Ayanian, 1994), this is not relevant to the present discussion of mortality rates.

Results of a survey in inner-city areas of Boston (Crawford et al., 1994) did not find black–white differences in *seeking* of care for cardiac symptoms (chest pain and shortness of breath) within a low social class area. Blacks were significantly less likely than whites to be referred to a cardiologist (as found in other studies), even when severity of symptoms and ability to pay were considered. Although this raises the possibility of racial biases in treatment recommendations, appropriateness of care received was not evaluated, and any impact on mortality rates is uncertain. Similar studies are needed among different metropolitan areas.

Higher death rates from kidney diseases in African Americans are well documented, including serious (or "end-stage") renal disease due to hypertension, diabetes mellitus, and certain other antecedent conditions. Even if survival rates after kidney transplantation were equal in blacks and whites, the higher incidence rates for various forms of renal disease in blacks than whites would result in higher mortality rates for blacks. Thus, prevention efforts including hypertension prevention and control, are needed among blacks. However, some of the black–white disparity in survival after kidney transplantation could be reduced by better care of black patients.

Longer waiting times by blacks than by whites for kidney transplantation reflect both the need for matching on HLA types and black–white differences in

HLA frequencies (mentioned in Chapter 2). The desire for matching of blood groups and tissue antigens (mainly HLA) is disadvantageous for blacks. In a study of 100 consecutive recipients of primary cadaveric renal transplants at the University of Mississippi Medical Center (1985–1991), HLA mismatching had no effect on graft survival among patients with private health insurance, and race had no additional effect after controlling for type of health insurance (i.e., Medicaid and Medicare vs. private commercial insurance) (Butkus et al., 1992). This suggests that universal health insurance coverage, along with other efforts to provide better care for black organ recipients with poor HLA matching, could help to improve the survival of black patients after transplantation. Apparently, studies have not been done comparing survival rates of black transplant patients living in different metropolitan areas. Social class of blacks, even those living in predominantly black (and high-poverty) areas, could modify treatment and prognosis.

After excluding renal diseases, elderly black Medicare enrollees were less likely than whites to receive 23 of 32 medical procedures or tests, even after some adjustment for financial barriers (Escarce et al., 1993). Physician decision-making processes for black patients may be relevant. In a nationally representative sample of hospitalized Medicare patients, quality of care was lower for patients who were black or came from poor neighborhoods within each category of hospital type. However, black patients were often treated at urban teaching hospitals, with higher quality care than rural or urban nonteaching hospitals. Therefore, overall quality of care and death rates did not differ between blacks and whites (Kahn et al., 1994). Studies are needed in adults under 65 years of age.

Evidence for better treatment at urban teaching hospitals could suggest that blacks in segregated inner cities may receive better care than blacks in other areas. Since whites living in the vicinity of such hospitals also could receive care (and better care than blacks), black–white differences in health care (and any effects on mortality) would occur in such urban areas. More detailed studies are needed of blacks and whites in areas near urban teaching hospitals, including consideration of transportation problems and attitudes and practices of physicians.

Studies of hospitalized patients do not include deaths of persons never hospitalized for various reasons, including death prior to reaching a hospital. Out-of-hospital cardiac arrest is a major factor in mortality from coronary heart disease. In Seattle, the age-adjusted annual incidence rate of such cardiac arrests in blacks was twice that of whites. While the difference was not due to response times of trained emergency teams (Cowie et al., 1993), neighborhood factors could have influenced delays in administering resuscitation by members of the community. The study was based on small numbers of events among blacks, because the Seattle MSA has a relatively small black population and relatively low black–white residential segregation. Comparative studies of blacks in MSAs that differ in segregation might be enlightening.

Finally, death rates from ill-defined causes are higher in blacks and other minorities than in whites. In classifications of diseases and causes of death, these causes are referred to as "symptoms, senility and ill-defined conditions". The differences are due in part to poorer access to care among blacks (Becker et al., 1990). Analysis of U.S. data showed that in 1978–1982 the age-adjusted rate of death from ill-defined causes for black males (41.3 per 100,000 per year) was more than three times that for white males (13.1 per 100,000), with a similar black/white ratio for females (25.0/7.6). Lack of health insurance and personal physician in remote rural areas, but also in inner cities, may be involved. Studies are needed of death rates from ill-defined conditions among blacks living in areas that differ by level of segregation.

Psychophysiologic Responses and Health

Discrimination is a cause of segregation, but it is not clear how the frequency and intensity of experiences with discrimination and racism by blacks vary with degree of segregation. Less contact with whites (as in segregated areas) also means less opportunity for direct experiences with discrimination. Also, the initial experiences of blacks moving out of segregated areas to less-segregated areas may involve encounters with discrimination and racism in relation to housing, bank loans, and other transactions. Moving into less segregated areas also could increase the perception (by blacks) of incongruity between high socioeconomic status and low social status due to dark skin color. Actual rates of exposure to discrimination and of specific types of responses to discrimination by blacks in relation to the level of residential segregation cannot be addressed in this review. As noted earlier, the discussion concerns the broader topic of the epidemiology of discrimination and racism rather than the epidemiology of American apartheid.

Discrimination and racism in relation to blood pressure
Studies on the physiologic effects of experiences with racial discrimination on the health of blacks have focused on the etiology of hypertension. The potential role of stress, involving the sympathetic nervous system, was mentioned in Chapter 2, with reference to the multidimensional nature of the race concept. In a study of 51 black and 50 white women 20–80 years old residing in Alameda County, CA, self-reported experience with racial discrimination was positively associated with the prevalence of self-reported high blood pressure among blacks (Krieger, 1989). The association did not reach statistical significance for the small sample size involved. However, women who stated that they usually kept quiet about unfair treatment (racism or discrimination) had a three-fold risk of high blood pressure compared with women who reported that they usually talked about and acted on such experiences.

Krieger (1989) hypothesized that acceptance of (or internalization of response to) discrimination was causally associated with higher blood pressure. The interview involved questions about feelings of unfair treatment, experiencing discrimination, or "being prevented from doing something" or "hassled" or "made to feel inferior" because of "race or color" at school, in getting a job, at work, in getting housing, in getting medical care and "from the police or in the courts" (Krieger, 1989). Studies are needed on the relationship between the frequency of, as well as the type of response to, such experiences among blacks according to level of residential segregation.

The experimental viewing of scenes depicting racist situations was associated with acute increases in measured blood pressure (Armstead et al., 1989) or heart rate (Jones et al., 1996) in samples of black college students. In view of Krieger's interpretation (1989), further studies should include assessment of reactions to such situations in terms of acceptance or denial of discrimination. In South Africa, a cohort or follow-up study of urbanized university students found that black students had greater levels of anxiety and suppressed anger than white students. Those black students who developed hypertension had significantly higher baseline levels of these variables than did those who did not develop hypertension. These factors, along with family instability, remained important in multivariate analyses of hypertension among black (but not white) students (Somova et al., 1995).

The prevalence of perceived discrimination among individual blacks should be documented in terms of specific time periods and entire lifetimes. In the National Health Access and Satisfaction Survey in 1992 (Blendon et al., 1995), racial discrimination during the past year was reported by one in seven blacks. This period prevalence rate (in epidemiologic terms) represents only the tip of the iceberg because the number of such events would increase if the time period were extended. The relationship between the frequency and intensity of these experiences and degree of segregation, and its interaction with social class among blacks, is apparently unknown.

Status incongruence

"Status incongruence" among blacks results from high social class lifestyle combined with low social status due to dark skin color (Dressler, 1993), which may be interpreted as resulting from discrimination. Degree of status incongruence was positively associated with blood pressure level and prevalence of hypertension among blacks in a small Alabama city, suggesting that "frequent frustrated social interactions" may lead to "autonomic arousal" and elevated blood pressure (Dressler, 1993, 1996). This situation may resemble that shown for demand–control aspects of the work environment in relation to cardiovascular reactivity and hypertension or heart disease (Kaufman et al., 1994). That is, lack of control over the work situation, but with high job demands for productivity, may be harmful to health.

The study of "status incongruence" among blacks is part of a broader area of research in medical sociology and epidemiology, dealing with "status inconsistency" in relation to health (Vernon and Buffler, 1988). Status inconsistency was first used to examine the detrimental effects of an individual's discrepancy in rankings on different hierarchies based on education, occupation, and income (i.e., measures of social class). The terminology used has varied, and different aspects of inconsistencies in status within an individual and pairs of individuals (e.g., spouses) have been emphasized by different investigators. Findings of studies on status inconsistency (variously defined) in relation to coronary heart disease risk have been mixed, with more consistency in findings among the limited number of studies on women than men (Vernon and Buffler, 1988).

The frequency of status incongruence among blacks living in different metropolitan areas, including those that differ in segregation, apparently has not been studied. Again, social class of blacks could be a modifying factor in both contributing to the likelihood of status incongruence and modulating its effects (Dressler, 1996).

Coping responses to stress
Sociological studies of stress have emphasized the limitations involved in examining only "life events" or acute stresses. Chronic strains and coping responses that mediate the impact of stresses may be more crucial with regard to health effects (Pearlin, 1989). Reactions to psychosocial stress in blacks could have health consequences, as discussed earlier with regard to discrimination (Krieger, 1989). "John Henryism," named after the black folk figure, involves hard-driving effort and active coping responses to psychosocial stressors (James et al., 1987; Weinrich et al., 1988). The questions involved in the John Henryism scale assess the degree of agreement with 12 statements that involve (for example) perceived control over one's life, ability to overcome obstacles and finish a job, and to "work even harder" when "things don't go the way [one] wants them to" (Weinrich et al., 1988). The first studies, in a predominantly rural area of North Carolina, showed higher mean (average) blood pressures among lower social class individuals scoring high on the John Henryism scale. In epidemiologic terms, there was an "interaction" between social class and the John Henryism score with regard to the outcome (hypertension). A similar study in a predominantly "middle-class" black population of North Carolina found that among persons with high John Henryism scores the prevalence of hypertension was only 15% in a higher social class stratum but reached 35% in a lower class group (James et al., 1987, 1992). Thus, the interaction was supported.

Regarding the John Henryism scale, lower class blacks may fare worse than higher class blacks (Figure 6-4), but the effects of residential segregation on the John Henryism score itself, and the strength of its association with hypertension, are unknown.

Coping may involve aspects of race and ethnicity other than those measured by the John Henryism scale. A study conducted with adolescents mainly in age groups prior to the appearance of the black–white difference in blood pressure levels found an association between lower systolic blood pressure and strong "African American self-concept" (AASC) in males, even after controlling for social class (parents' education) and body mass index (weight divided by height) (Scribner et al., 1995). However, the AASC scale (see Chapter 2) used in this study was admittedly crude and somewhat unreliable so that further studies are needed.

Black communities with high rates of poverty and social isolation (or residential segregation) may have high prevalences of low "perceived self-efficacy" due to economic marginality and other adverse aspects of life in hypersegregated

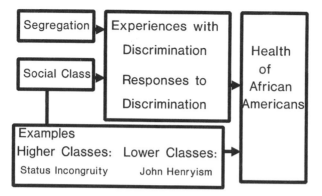

Figure 6-4. Social class, segregation, and effects on black health.

areas (Wilson, 1991a,b) (Chapter 3). Both individual and community levels of ethnic identification and perceived control or efficacy should be studied in relation to responses to discrimination and other stresses and in relation to hypertension and other health-related outcomes.

Hostility
Studies on the association between "hostility" and coronary artery disease have been inconsistent (Barefoot et al., 1995; Helmer et al., 1991), although hostility in late adolescence may be predictive of risk factors later in life (Siegler et al., 1992). More recently, in a study of Danish adults (aged 50 years in 1964) followed up until 1991, hostility scale scores were associated with increased risks of myocardial infarction (about 50% increase) and total mortality (about 44%) in statistical models that controlled for other risk factors (Barefoot et al., 1995). The hostility scale incorporated items described as "cynicism" or negative beliefs about the "trustworthiness" of others, "hostile attribution" items or suspicion of harmful intent by others, "hostile" affect or mood, and the endorsement of being aggressive or "rough" in solving problems related to the behavior of others. The scale used appeared to be highly stable or repeatable over time. Items from this hostility scale had been used previously in a cross-sectional or prevalence study of 5,115 black and white young adults (18–30 years old) in four large U.S. urban areas (Scherwitz et al., 1992). Higher levels of hostility were associated with various unhealthy habits including smoking of tobacco and marijuana, increased alcohol consumption, and greater dietary intake of calories (but not percentage of calories from fat).

Although cross-sectional studies are difficult to interpret in terms of causality, these findings provide a potential (at least partial) explanation for the positive findings of some studies on hostility and mortality from coronary heart disease. The findings were consistent by race, as well as age, sex, and education level. Previous studies had been restricted in terms of racial and educational composition of participants. Interestingly, findings from prospective studies were interpreted as suggesting that hostile persons may have used food, cigarettes, and marijuana as part of a coping response to stress and low levels of social support.

Other stresses and responses, conclusions, and research needs
As shown by a study in the San Francisco–Oakland area using an "abbreviated hassles index," stressful environments may contribute to cigarette smoking among urban African Americans (Romano et al., 1991). Smoking has adverse effects on immune responses. There is also increasing interest in the effects on stresses on the immune system, with consequences for health, including both infectious and chronic diseases (Ader et al., 1995). Such effects could be relevant to variation in the health of blacks by neighborhood characteristics (including degree of segregation).

An explorative ethnographic study of factors perceived by black women 25–75 years old in three sororities to be important in obesity suggested that occupational stressors related to racism (and sexism) should be examined, as well as overall perceived stress (Walcott-McQuigg, 1995). Future research should consider the possible interactions between variables (discrimination experiences, John Henryism score, social class, occupation, and AASC) in relation to risk factors or conditions other than blood pressure or hypertension, such as obesity, smoking, and use of alcohol and other drugs. Degree of residential segregation also could interact with these variables in complex ways (Fig. 6-4). The prevalences of the factors discussed in this section (i.e., status incongruence, high scores on the John Henryism scale, and hostility) have not been examined among blacks living in areas that differ in degree of segregation. Research into psychological and psychophysiologic responses to discrimination and racism should consider the life experiences association with segregation.

The studies reviewed in this section suggest that discrimination and racism may have complex associations with hypertension in that the responses of black individuals appear to be more important than exposure to discrimination. The association between high John Henryism scores and high blood pressure in black men only within lower social classes could indicate that resources available to persons of higher social class may reduce the hypertensive effects of discrimination. Higher class blacks may experience a lower level of "frustration" or discrimination (Scribner et al., 1995) but higher "status incongruence" (with uncertain effects on health).

Community-wide studies are needed on the prevalence of stresses and responses to these stresses (e.g., immunologic and hormonal) in relation to the prevalence of specific diseases in blacks. Ongoing longitudinal studies of mortality in large national samples of the U.S. population (Chapter 4) could modify their protocols to include administration of questionnaires on stresses, hostility, social support, and coping mechanisms, along with their interactions with levels of social class and segregation.

Housing and Neighborhood Quality

Other aspects of the quality of environment in segregated areas (including urban ghettos) that could influence health include crowding, safety of neighborhoods with regard to crime, injury, and homicide, exposure to noise and other stressors such as various types of environmental pollution and occupational hazards, and degree of access to recreational facilities for leisure-time physical activity. Some of these conditions were mentioned with reference to the concentration or neighborhood effects of the combination of high poverty rates among blacks and black–white segregation (Chapter 3).

A few housing indexes used as independent variables in multiple regression analyses were significant predictors of nonwhite age-adjusted death rates in Kitagawa and Hauser's analyses (1973) of death rates in 1960. The degree of segregation was not considered. In Chapter 5, the segregation index was (as anticipated) correlated strongly with housing and neighborhood quality variables among the 33 large MSAs used in the analysis of homicide rates and neighborhood quality in relation to mortality in young adult black men. Low self-reported ratings of neighborhood quality by black householders made some contribution to the prediction of mortality rates for 15–44-year-old black males in 33 MSAs, but the results did not reach statistical significance when segregation index was included in the regression model (Chapter 5). This indicates that the association between segregation index and mortality cannot be entirely explained by the association between segregation and the crude index of neighborhood quality. These analyses involved such limited data on neighborhood quality for blacks that they can only suggest the need for further studies.

The remainder of this discussion considers specific aspects of quality of life for blacks in inner cities that might be considered by studies in the area of the epidemiology of American apartheid.

Crowding and urban decay

The potential impact of crowding on health has long been of interest to epidemiologists and public health researchers. While inner city areas may decline in total population, crowing may persist, especially in public housing projects (Chapter 2). "Overcrowding" or high population density is related to the spread of various infectious diseases including tuberculosis and measles (Aaby et al., 1984). Associations have also been reported with chronic diseases. The potential mechanisms, other than increased exposure to infectious agents involved in some cancers, are uncertain.

A number of specific cancers were associated with population density (persons per square mile) independently of social class in an ecologic study of cancer incidence rates using census-tract indicators (Baquet et al., 1991). Overcrowding in the home during childhood has been associated with high rates of stomach cancer in England and Wales, suggesting the role of transmission of agents such as the microorganisms known to be involved in gastritis and stomach cancer (Barker et al., 1990). Thus, degree of crowding should be included in ecologic studies examining the association between segregation and the health of blacks. Studies in areas with large public housing developments might be useful.

The deterioration of minority neighborhoods in parts of New York City after about 1974 was associated with temporal increases in death rates for tuberculosis (Wallace and Wallace, 1990). There also was a rise in homicides and drug-related deaths in New York City after 1978 associated with the occurrence of "contagious urban decay and disruption of social networks. No data were given on time trends in black–white segregation. The deterioration in the quality of the environment, along with rationing of health care (Wallace, 1990), could have contributed to increases in tuberculosis mortality rates in parts of New York City. A reversal in the trend for tuberculosis in New York City occurred from 1988 to 1993. Various public health measures, including strategies to increase patient compliance with therapy at municipal tuberculosis clinics, may have contributed to this decline (Frankel, 1994) (see Chapter 7).

Prevalence and mortality rates for another lung disease, asthma, are higher in urban than rural areas in the United States. In Philadelphia, census tracts with a high proportion of blacks in the population tended to have higher total death rates from asthma in poor but not in more affluent areas. This suggested the importance of overcrowding, low-quality housing, and low level of education. These potential "mediators" of the neighborhood effects of segregation are probably related to more specific risk factors such as exposure to dust-mite and cockroach allergens. Also mentioned were a constellation of potentially contributing factors including "level of physical decay" of housing and neighborhoods, crime, illicit drug use, family nondysfunction, hopelessness, and despair (Lang and Polansky, 1994). This constellation of quality-of-life factors in Philadelphia resembles those described around the turn of the century by Du Bois in *The Philadelphia Negro* (1899).

Opportunities for participating in safe leisure-time physical activity may be reduced in inner-city areas where blacks predominate. Such barriers could help to explain lower levels of activity among blacks relative to whites, especially in women, after adjustment for income level, and could play a role in black–white differences in the prevalence of obesity (Kumanyika, 1987; Washburn et al., 1992). Surveys of public housing residents (more than 90% African American and predominantly women) in Birmingham indicated that a sedentary lifestyle was more common than in white middle-class areas, although poorer health status (rather than lack of safe facilities) was a factor (Lewis et al., 1993). Comparative studies of different public housing projects are needed, as often mentioned in this book.

The urban underclass may be especially vulnerable to death during heat waves, an underestimated cause of death in the United States (Kalkstein, 1995). Cities in the East and Midwest have the largest numbers of heat-related deaths, where buildings in ghettos in St. Louis, Chicago, and New York are especially unsuited to hot conditions. This writer is unaware of any statistics on the racial and neighborhood distributions of decedents during heat waves, such as those that occurred in Chicago and other cities during the summer of 1995.

Tobacco and illicit drugs
An example of research on health-related behavior among blacks in public housing projects may illustrate the effects of concentration of poverty. Black–white differences in smoking behavior include lower rates of cessation among blacks. Among young black women residing in subsidized public housing in Chicago, characteristics unfavorable to smoking cessation were found (Man-

fredi et al., 1992). Further studies of health-related behaviors are needed among black residents of public housing projects.

Another aspect of life in predominantly poor and minority neighborhoods in inner cities is greater exposure to advertising of tobacco and alcohol products. In San Diego, for example, point-of-purchase advertisements of tobacco products were more common in African-American communities than in white or Hispanic communities (Wildey et al., 1992). Advertisements in liquor stores and independent markets were especially common (Woodruff et al., 1995).

In a metropolitan area (i.e., Chicago) much more highly segregated than San Diego, a survey was conducted of 5,924 billboards in two groups of wards (16 predominantly white and 34 predominantly minority). The study was done in response to reports by community groups and local newspaper accounts of unlicensed billboards advertising tobacco and alcohol. Minority wards were found to have almost three times as many billboards advertising tobacco as white wards; the means were 36 and 13 per ward. The difference was even larger for billboards advertising alcohol (Hackbarth et al., 1995). In another analysis, a statistically significant positive correlation was found between the percentage of minority residents in a ward and the occurrence of billboards advertising tobacco or alcohol. Community groups in Chicago are attempting to use these data in campaigns to remove unlicensed billboards and ban advertising of tobacco products on billboards, in Chicago public transit, and in Chicago sports stadiums (Hackbarth et al., 1995).

Tobacco and alcohol are "gateway" drugs that lead to illicit drug use by adolescents. In an intensive interview study in 1984–1986 of about 2,500 teenage medical patients in 10 programs involving health clinics (based in communities or schools), about one-third of youths (predominantly black and female) were likely to become involved in regular substance abuse. Regular tobacco use influenced the progression to substance abuse in both male and female patients (Earls and Powell, 1988). The importance of neighborhood effects on cocaine use is mentioned in Chapter 3.

Environmental exposure to hazardous substances
Black–white disparities in exposure to hazardous substances in the occupational environment have been shown (Robinson, 1989) but also need to be examined by census tract or smaller areas. A national surveillance system of death rates related to occupational injuries showed higher rates for blacks than whites in each year from 1980 to 1989, although the death rates declined more for blacks than whites (Stout et al., 1996). Mining, construction, transportation, and public utilities industries were associated with the highest death rates, but data were not presented by geographic area or urban versus rural residence of decedents. Some 82% of workplace homicides occurred in connection with robberies or other crimes, which suggests possible differences in homicide rates by neighborhood of workplace, but studies are needed on place of residence in relation to place of work.

Blacks in certain inner-city areas are exposed more often than whites to various toxic environmental hazards. Excessive lead exposure in inner-city black children (Johnson and Coulberson, 1993), while mainly relevant to intelligence and physical–neurologic development, also may be relevant to kidney diseases (and hence mortality) in blacks. The role of racism has been suggested with regard to the placement of toxic waste-disposal sites near communities where minorities predominate (Anon., 1994; Bryant and Mohai, 1992; Johnson and Coulberson, 1993). These differences in exposure may have limited impact on black–white differences in death rates, but a need to enhance databases of demographics of communities with such sites has been recognized.

Community organizations were apparently effective in altering waste disposal patterns in Houston (Bullard, 1983). This is an example of the role of community empowerment in modulating neighborhood or concentration effects (Fig. 6-2). Enhanced political power in more highly segregated black communities could act as a buffer against any deleterious health effects of living in such areas (LaVeist, 1992, 1993), as discussed earlier in this chapter. Community-based primary-care health centers, often located in predominantly minority inner-city areas, can be a catalyst for various community activities such as improving the physical environment (Chapter 7). Future ecologic studies of the association between degree of segregation and mortality rates in young adults should include data on the number of community health centers and the number of black clients served in each MSA, along with detailed information on the medical services provided.

Conclusions and Research Needs

Racism has been called the "missing variable" in studies of racial–ethnic differences in health (Smith and Egger, 1992). This chapter has shown that ecologic studies of the association between mortality and segregation (which is largely due to discrimination) are needed involving geographic units smaller than cities or MSAs. Cause-specific mortality analyses for blacks should be included. Also needed are studies aimed at explaining the relatively low mortality of blacks living in certain less-segregated urban areas, especially in certain California MSAs, in the past (for infant mortality) or in the latest years studied (for young adult blacks).

Within hypersegregated MSAs, black mortality rates in census tracts or block groups (Chapter 2) should be studied. These "small-area" studies could include analyses of death rates among blacks in census tracts or block groups with unusually high proportions of blacks in the population, taking into account the black poverty rate in each area. Because of statistical instability of death rates for individual small areas, areas with similar characteristics could be combined. While each small area would be more homogeneous in social class than larger units (such as MSAs), the possibility of region-specific effects, or local factors peculiar to a neighborhood, could be difficult to address.

Conclusions derived from ecologic studies using small areas, especially block groups, regarding associations between social class and health may not differ from those obtained by studies of individuals (Krieger, 1992). However, future studies on segregation and social class in relation to health outcomes could use "hybrid" study designs. These studies combine ecologic data on rates of disease or death by geographic area with surveys of *individuals* in these specific geographic units. The analyses could include "exposure" variables that are ecologic or "structural," such as the proportion of blacks in the census tract, as well as survey data on histories of segregation and discrimination among individuals. "Hybrid" study designs may be attractive if survey information on quality of life and neighborhood can be piggybacked on existing surveys and combined with data on death rates by groups of census tracts. Because surveys are costly, even when added as special supplements to existing surveys, studies may include only a limited number of selected MSAs. MSAs selected may be similar in socioeconomic characteristics for blacks (or in black/white ratios of these characteristics) but differ in segregation and mortality rates. Neighborhood factors, as assessed by surveys, could be studied in relation to variation in mortality rates.

Due to the limitations of ecologic studies, longitudinal or cohort epidemiologic studies of blacks should obtain personal histories of social class indicators, experiences with discrimination, and psychological reactions to discrimination. Data on segregation indexes and "mediator" variables related to the quality of environment of residential areas (past and present) should be obtained as potential "risk factors" for disease and death. Such studies could benefit from collaboration between epidemiologists and both social and behavioral scientists. Longitudinal studies also could evaluate the potential applicability of an effect similar to the "drift" hypothesis or "reverse causal path" studied in relation to the association between income level and mortality (mentioned in Chapter 4). With reference to residential segregation, the selective migration of healthier black persons from highly segregated areas could affect mortality rates within these areas. It is more difficult to envision migration of less healthy blacks into segregated areas (perhaps to seek medical care at urban teaching hospitals).

Further studies are needed on trends in and factors associated with discrimination and segregation and on the physiologic pathways whereby discrimination might influence physical and mental health. Discrimination and racism may have effects on the health of blacks independent of any effects of segregation (Figs. 1-1 and 6-3). The role of racism in health care is receiving increasing attention by medical anthropologists, as witnessed by a special issue of *Medical Anthropology Quarterly* (Vol. 7, pp. 323–402) in 1994 (see also Harrison, 1994, 1995).

Hypersegregated MSAs have continued to have high black infant mortality rates in the 1980s and early 1990s, and the segregation index has continued to be a significant predictor of variation in black mortality rates for young adult males (15–44 years old) among large MSAs (Chapter 5). Future studies should include analyses of cause-specific death rates for blacks living in areas that differ in degree of segregation. The occurrence of relatively low mortality rates in infants and young adults in certain metropolitan areas, although affected by statistical instability due to small population sizes, suggests that health inequalities can be achieved even in the absence of equality in social class. However, the overall quality of life for blacks versus whites in these areas is another issue.

Table 6-3 summarizes some issues in the epidemiology of American apart-

Table 6-3. Some factors to be considered in multidimensional studies of the epidemiology of disease in blacks and whites

Socio-cultural dimension	Biologic–genetic dimension
Ethnicity and acculturation	Genetics and admixture
Degree of acculturation	Degree of white admixture
	Group measures
	Individual measures
Specific ethnic subgroups (e.g., specific Caribbean immigrant groups; generations of ancestors in the United States)	Genetic correlates of subgroup membership and self-identification
Degree of identification with "black" ethnicity	
Social class variables	
Status incongruence	Psychophysiologic responses (biochemical, physiologic)
Experiences with discrimination and segregation	
Residential segregation	
Quality of life and environment	Specific biologic responses, including immune function,
Housing and neighborhood quality	pulmonary function, biomarkers of exposure to toxic agents, carcinogens

heid and in the broader area of the epidemiology of discrimination and racism. Most desirable would be longitudinal studies including early-life factors and a chronicle of experiences with segregation and discrimination, as well as reactions to these experiences. All effects of segregation need not be detrimental, because segregation may promote group cohesion, solidarity, and political power. However, perceived self-esteem and self-efficacy may be adversely affected by isolation from the mainstream economy and society (Wilson, 1987, 1991a,b). Actual levels of experience with discrimination need to be quantified for blacks according to level of segregation.

The multidimensional view of race and ethnicity (Chapter 2) includes consideration of differences in biologic characteristics and genetic markers (Table 6-3). Variation in degree of white admixture *within* black populations residing in different geographic areas, with different levels of segregation, also could be considered in multidisciplinary studies of specific diseases in relation to the multidimensional nature of "race" (Chapter 2).

Future ecologic studies should include information on quality of life for blacks and whites in inner cities of MSAs. Another area of research relevant to the epidemiology of American apartheid that should be expanded is "urban anthropology." Research areas of interest include the health effects of migration from rural to urban areas and neighborhood effects in urban areas on culture (including gang membership, illicit drug use, and the "business" of illicit drug sale), quality of life, and attitudes about out-of-wedlock births. The need for comparative studies on quality of life, health, and health care of blacks living in housing projects in different cities or MSAs is mentioned in Chapter 7, on social and health policy issues.

7

Some Issues in Social
and Health Policies

An editorial in *The Lancet* discussing the "underclass" in both England and the United States suggested that "compassion and public policy" once attempted "through such activities as the new deal and the welfare state" to attack the underclass but that declining faith in this viewpoint may be "inflating" the underclass (Anon., 1990). It was also suggested that a "walk about in London" would bring "shame and indignation" regarding the plight of the "underclass." Similar sentiments would be evoked by a visit to many large U.S. cities, especially the older metropolises in parts of the North and Midwest where blacks migrated in large numbers during the early to middle twentieth century.

After visiting London's East End slums, white progressive reformers in Philadelphia around the turn of the twentieth century sponsored Du Bois' research to diagnose and explain the social disease. Sweden was used as an antithetical model (Lewis, 1993). Du Bois' *The Philadelphia Negro* (1899) painted a grim portrait of the quality of life of many urban blacks, a situation that has endured and even worsened (Massey and Denton, 1993).

Sweden was used as model for New Dealers and more recently with regard to approaches to the problem of infant mortality (Najman, 1993; Hogue and Hargreaves, 1993). However, Latin-American refugees in Sweden have higher rates of self-reported illness independent of social class and education, probably reflecting "social degradation and a sense of discrimination" resulting from "xenophobia" or fear of foreigners (Sundquist, 1995). An underprivileged social and health status awaits new immigrants.

In the United States, the "underprivileged" status of the black population in terms of mortality rates (Kitagawa and Hauser, 1973) persists (Chapter 4), especially in the most highly segregated metropolitan areas (Chapter 5). The tentative conclusion is that the problem of the concentration of blacks in high-poverty areas due to segregation, with its effects on quality of life and health, must be addressed. If the segregation that causes such concentration of blacks is **127** not addressed, the quality of life and quality of health care in segregated inner cities (occupied predominantly by minorities) could be targeted.

McCord and Freeman's stark portrayal of life expectancy and death rates in Harlem (1990), described as comparable (in terms of needs) to a federal "disaster area" or a developing country (Bangladesh), also mentioned a similar situation in Philadelphia. These findings did not precipitate a response in any way comparable to those associated with acute natural disasters. The Carter Administration's Harlem Health Task Force, created in 1976, recommended expansion of community clinics, drug treatment centers, and community outreach programs, but funding was limited, and no decline in death rates from 1960 to 1980 was found by McCord and Freeman (1990). These approaches do not deal with segregation itself, but with its consequences on quality of life and health.

In an assessment of the role of epidemiology in health policy, Kuller (1988) noted that "the critical challenge" was "to narrow the socioeconomic gradient in morbidity and mortality." The mortality gradient has been increasing in many western countries due to increasing inequalities in the distribution of income and education within these countries (Chapters 3 and 4). In public health there is lack of agreement on the need to attack poverty (or low-income) itself or to continue to develop interventions aimed at reducing the public health impact of persistent poverty and insufficient income. A similar situation occurs with regard to the question of whether segregation itself or its effects on the health of blacks should be targeted in developing social and health policies.

First, the choice between addressing poverty or its effects on health are discussed briefly, followed by consideration of the similar dichotomy of attacking segregation or the associated health issues for blacks in inner cities. With regard to the latter alternative, some examples of community-based public health programs in Harlem and other hypersegregated areas will be mentioned.

Addressing Poverty and Segregation

Attacking Poverty, Including Urban Black Poverty

An editorial in the *American Journal of Public Health* referred not only to Sweden (with its expanded welfare system) but also to American history in recognizing the need to attack poverty itself. The progressive child welfare movement in America, inspired by F. Kelly and other women, resulted in improvements in health "through reducing poverty" and "ameliorating the effects of poverty on the poor" (Hogue and Hargreaves, 1993).

One analyst of cross-national data concluded that

> using the welfare system to more effectively reduce the income gap between rich and poor, supported by a renewed emphasis on the education system to educate the poor and retrain the unemployed, appears to be the only way of producing a substantial reduction in socioeconomic inequalities in mortality. (Najman 1993, p. 165)

The situation may be more complex. The underclass may be (in part) a symptom of the deeper economic problem of a periodically "unemployable" segment of society even if job training programs prove successful. This reflects such trends as foreign market competition and rapid technological changes (Gans, 1993). A modernized version of the New Deal, an unpopular idea in the 1980s and 1990s, has been advocated, especially for poverty areas and ghettos (as defined in Chapter 3). "Unemployable" persons were recognized in New Deal national programs, especially after state governments were found indifferent and/or ill-equipped to handle them (Leuchtenburg, 1963; McElvaine, 1993; Rank, 1994).

The vagaries of sociopolitical attitudes regarding federal (or federal–state) public assistance programs are obvious. The compassionate viewpoint espoused in the *Lancet* editorial (Anon., 1990) mentioned earlier regarding the "welfare state" may not be shared by the majority of American citizens in the 1990s. Many conservatives continue to view "welfare," or certain public assistance programs such as AFDC, as remnants of failed federal government approaches and as "causes" of social problems, thus rejecting expansion (or even retention) of programs targeted to the poor (Murray, 1984).

For those who do not reject public assistance programs, the debate is over the proper balance between programs "targeted" to the poor and "universal" approaches that also benefit the nonpoor (e.g., Darby, 1996; Greenstein, 1991; Jencks and Peterson, 1991). With regard to blacks (including those in ghettos), targeting with federally sponsored antipoverty programs has not been considered politically realistic by some sociologists (Wilson, 1987; Gans, 1993). Extension and expansion of the earned income tax credit, which is not viewed as a "liberal" program, may be a more realistic goal than expansion of public assistance programs, especially for blacks. As part of a "new war on poverty," even "conservatives" have advocated or developed programs to address the economic problems of inner cities through such efforts as enterprise zones and resident management and tenant ownership of public housing (Kelso, 1994; Darby, 1996). These programs are targeted to low-income persons (disproportionately black) or high-poverty inner-city areas. The Department of Housing and Urban Development (HUD), although often targeted for abolition, provides assistance to about 1 million households consisting of single women with children, or about 25% of all low-income subsidized households (more than half of which are classified as black) (Weicher, 1996).

The generation of jobs by investment in "infrastructure" has been proposed for decaying inner cities and "social investment" in "older urban areas" (Rosen, 1995) affected by relocation of industries, often without attention to the ensuing "social burdens." This situation was emphasized in W.J. Wilson's "spatial mismatch" model of the problems of inner cities (1987, 1991a,b). In discussing concentration or neighborhood effects (Chapter 3), the "structural" problems of ghetto poverty were noted to include lack of opportunities for new businesses. In many large inner cities, including not only the hypersegregated MSAs of the Northeast and Midwest but also Los Angeles, black neighborhoods have benefitted least from urban economic development, and the priority of improving black housing and neighborhoods has received little attention. Private sector jobs have failed to grow fast enough, and discriminatory employment practices have persisted (Peterson, 1994). Obviously, the needs far outstrip the capacities of such efforts as enterprise zones.

Attacking Segregation and Discrimination

Enterprise zones and public housing ownership issues do not address segregation, but rather some of its effects on quality of life. Programs to move tenants from inner-city public housing to suburban areas (Chapter 2) do address segregation. Segregation is part of the problem of the "colour line," or racial discrimination in the face of "high ideals" of "justice" (W.E.B. Du Bois, quoted by Lewis, 1993, p. 251). America's right to have "moral weight" in the world was later challenged, by (for example) J. Baldwin (1963), G. Myrdal (1944), and sociologist H. Gans (1993). The problems of the "color line" will persist and grow in the twenty-first century. By the year 2050, non-Hispanic whites are projected to comprise 56% of the population (a bare majority), with 16% of black and 23% of Hispanic origin (Day, 1993). In economic downturns blacks have fared worse than whites. The black and Hispanic "underclasses" may grow in numbers (Massey, 1993; Massey and Denton, 1993).

In attacking social inequalities (including poverty rates) involving blacks, Allport (1969) concluded that prejudice was too difficult and deep-seated to be addressed successfully, although opinions may have changed somewhat (Ponterotto and Pederson, 1993). Segregation itself, as one manifestation of prejudice and discrimination, has proved persistent, presumably because the underlying causes (Chapter 2) have not been aggressively addressed.

However, programs aimed at removing ghettos from America have been advocated (Fuchs, 1993; Lemann, 1992; Steinberg, 1989). In attempting to contrast his view with W.J. Wilson's "universalist" or "race-neutral" approaches to poverty among blacks, Steinberg (1989) recommended a national program to eliminate ghettos through urban reconstruction programs that involve empowering local groups without ignoring the "racial and cultural dimensions" of the underclass.

Reformers aiming at "slum" clearance had limited success in the New Deal because of vested interest groups such as real estate associations, insurance companies, and building trade unions. President Roosevelt directed that political-legislative accommodations be made to these industries (Leuchtenburg, 1963). M.L. King Jr.'s "End Slums" campaign in Chicago in 1965 was regarded as too vague and grandiose (especially in Chicago) by other advisors. A series of marches in white neighborhoods in Chicago was greeted by violent responses, and a riot occurred in the West Side ghetto (Lemann, 1992). The legacy of the open-housing plan reached between King and the Mayor of Chicago in 1965 is a program that moved small numbers of blacks "one by one" (selected from many applicants) from the housing projects to the suburbs. The history of slum clearance and "urban renewal" has been described elsewhere (Fuchs, 1990; Gans, 1993; Massey and Denton, 1993; Quadagno, 1994).

Housing voucher systems have been advocated to replace high-density public housing (Massey and Denton, 1993). In 1995, the federal government (HUD) announced a takeover of housing projects in Chicago, with the intention of dispersal of their occupants. Even if increased use of "scattered housing" and housing vouchers for low-income blacks could be achieved, the availability of low-income housing could decline. The Chicago Housing Authority's chairman wanted, in Vergara's words (1995), to "deconcentrate poor people" not only by building more scatter-site housing of mixed-income groups (thus reducing segregation by social class and race) but also by changing the social class mixture of residents of the "infamous" Cabrini-Green development. These efforts would be paid for by a combination of federal and private investment.

Historically, efforts with housing vouchers for low-income persons have been minimal. In the "fair housing" initiative in Yonkers, NY, only 200 units were built (Massey and Denton, 1993). Sociologist H.J. Gans (1993) has argued that "private enterprise" did little about housing for the poor after the federal government ended construction of low-income public housing during the second Nixon administration (around 1970) (Table 2-3). One lesson from the history of "urban renewal" is that there must be viable alternative residences for people displaced from low-income public housing projects.

Extensive programs based on voucher systems as a replacement for high-density public housing projects would encounter the problem of white rejection, when the proportion of blacks in specific neighborhoods exceeds a certain threshold (Chapter 2). In Boston, it has been alleged that "the same ugly, racially charged resistance" seen 20 to 30 years ago has emerged in response to efforts to integrate blacks into white-occupied public housing (Ray, 1995). Unfortunately, the maximum extent of such efforts as the Gatreaux Project in Chicago is often limited to near tokenism due to opposition and reactions (including moving out) by residents of predominantly white neighborhoods (Chapter 2). Movement of blacks is often restricted to areas close to the ghettos (Vergara, 1995). Small numbers of black families moved to low-income suburban units, as in Houston, where protests from the Ku Klux Klan were planned (*Los Angeles Times*, January 14, 1994). Noteworthy was the fact that federal intervention from HUD was required in attempting to overcome failures of local housing authorities to counteract years of segregation in public housing complexes.

The need to plan for alternative low-income housing must be emphasized in decisions regarding the future of such developments. However, the basic dilemma concerns balancing the effort given to improving the quality of life and health for black residents of "better" housing projects and that devoted to dismantling other projects as a hindrance to the increased integration desired by the majority of blacks. Minimally, anthropological and sociological studies are needed comparing quality of life in various public housing projects, such as those in East Harlem (Freidenberg, 1995; Williams and Kornblum, 1995).

Greater enforcement of existing legislation against discrimination in housing would be required to reduce segregation (Massey and Denton, 1993). This also holds for the 1964 Civil Rights Act dealing with segregation of health care facilities; expanded legislation has been proposed (Watson, 1994). Institutional racism includes subtle and sometimes unintentional discrimination in health care (King, 1996), as discussed in Chapter 6. Educational programs in schools and colleges dealing with racism would be needed to attempt to address prejudice and discrimination or the initial phases of the causal chains shown in Figures 1-1, 6-2, and 6-3.

Addressing the Health Effects of Poverty and Segregation

Another view of health inequalities by income or social class (irrespective of race and ethnicity) urges concentration on addressing the effects of poverty and low income on health rather than the income inequalities themselves. According to this view, the

> damaging effects of poverty on healthful child development can be ameliorated without invoking politically troubling schemes of income redistribution, desirable as they might be. (Miller, 1992)

It has been argued that the biological causes of diseases associated with poverty and crowding can be overcome by public health (for example, immunization and nutritional programs) as well as improved medical treatment. Therefore, the persistence of inequities in income, both within each race and between races, could lose their importance with regard to public health (Holtzman, 1995; Weatherall, 1995).

Disparities in health insurance coverage between whites and minorities (blacks and Hispanics) are largely due to differences in social class (Chapter 3). If "income redistribution" (Miller, 1992) is avoided, health care access and quality of care issues would need more attention. In "The Defeat of Health Care Reform: Misplaced Mistrust of Government," Feingold (1995) mentioned not only the plight of the "working poor" but also high poverty rates among African Americans and Hispanics as important factors in inequalities in health that health care reform itself will not cure. How much of the "effects of poverty" on health (Miller, 1992) would be overcome by such efforts as expanded primary care access for underserved groups is not clear.

However, the "perinatal paradox" (mentioned in Chapter 1) illustrates the limits of the medical model. Universal health insurance and medical technological advances cannot solve all problems of inequities in health outcomes because of the harmful underlying social conditions of the neighborhoods in which the surviving infants (and children and adults) must live (Chapter 3).

The dichotomy between antipoverty and public health or medical intervention programs is itself difficult to maintain, because some public assistance programs provide assistance relevant to health care and health status. Coverage of low-income persons is incomplete for programs such as Head Start, WIC, and AFDC, as evident both in official reports from the Bureau of the Census and in population surveys (Chapter 3). Relatively small proportions of the low-income population (regardless of race) receive support from multiple "safety net" programs (Medicaid, food stamps, and AFDC) (Chapter 3), despite the evidence for beneficial effects on health-related outcomes such as nutrition, child development, and birth outcomes for high-risk women (Chapter 6). Miller (1992) asked what would happen to the health of children if existing programs such as Head Start were "financed and implemented at levels sufficient for the assessed need." Head Start is far from a universal program (Lemann, 1991; Zigler et al., 1994). This is even more true for Healthy Start (Chapter 6), initiated in 1991 as an infant mortality reduction program involving 15 sites with exceptionally high infant mortality rates, including several hypersegregated metropolitan areas.

The same argument about addressing the health outcomes associated with poverty rather than poverty or low income itself can be applied to discrimination and segregation. If discrimination, including discrimination in housing (which causes segregation), is not addressed as an underlying factor in black poverty and the concentration of blacks in high-poverty areas in order to reduce the high death rates for blacks in hypersegregated areas, then public health programs that reach blacks in these areas must be intensified in order to improve health status and survival. Of course, poor health status or higher death rates for blacks are not the only rationale for attacking black ghetto poverty.

Although not actually examined, inadequate health care was regarded as having such an obvious role in explaining the very high mortality rates for young adult black men in Harlem that public health workers were urged to move directly toward "lobbying" for interventions (McCord and Freeman, 1990). Presumably, this would emphasize improving access to primary-care physicians in Harlem.

While targeting public health programs to blacks has been advocated by leaders in medicine and public health (e.g., DeVita, 1985; Freeman, 1993), the issue is controversial. Some argue that such programs should target the poor or low-income persons rather than minorities (including those living in ghettos) because of the greater public health impact on the total population. However, the high total infant mortality rate in America relative to many other industrialized countries is due in part to the persistently high infant mortality rates in blacks (Singh and Yu, 1995), especially those living in hypersegregated metropolitan areas (Chapter 5). Whatever the explanation for higher death rates among black infants and young adults in hypersegregated urban areas, these populations can be targeted with public health programs.

Although ghettos have not been specifically targeted, national planning eforts in public health have involved specific targets or objectives for blacks. *Healthy People 2000* (U.S. Department of Health and Human Services, 1991) included not only national objectives for all racial and ethnic groups combined but also specific objectives for specific minority groups, such as infant mortality rates for blacks (Chapter 5). The importance of "looking beyond the aggregate data" and considering "special population groups" (minorities) has been emphasized, because the overall evaluation of the success of the national effort is "compromised" by such closer examination.

Preliminary analyses of the 300 objectives showed that the number of objectives for which the trend was in the "wrong direction" was considerably higher for minorities than for the total population (McGinnis and Lee, 1995). For blacks, asthma, adolescent pregnancies, AIDS incidence, and homicides were increasingly diverging from the Year 2000 targets. These problems are especially important for blacks living in inner cities (and especially in ghettos). Although the adverse quality of life, health, and safety effects of high-density housing projects would appear obvious, more epidemiologic research appears to be needed. Epidemiologic studies of the causes of violence suggest the importance of exposure to violence by black adolescents in high-crime areas, along with personal characteristics such as feelings of hopelessness and depression (DuRant et al., 1994). These problems are prevalent in ghettos (Chapter 3).

While *Healthy People 2000* included specific target objectives for blacks, specific programs targeted to blacks and minorities were not addressed. *Healthy Communities 2000: Model Standards* presented guidelines for health agencies working with community leaders and "representatives of affected populations." Minority groups were not specifically mentioned, but assessing community "power structures" was part of the process (American Public Health Association, 1991). There has been a movement toward inclusion of black community leaders and groups in planning and conducting public health interventions. Some examples are now discussed, with special reference to blacks in inner cities.

Public Health Programs in Black Communities and Ghettos

The 1992 National Health Access and Satisfaction Survey oversampled households with annual incomes of $20,000 or less. Among the 1,987 households (1,337 with low income), blacks rated the adequacy or quality of health care, along with education and police services, in the community lower than did whites (Blendon et al., 1995). Geographic areas or communities known to contain large numbers of poor blacks can be targeted with efforts to improve medical care and public health interventions.

In a survey of 1,196 black leaders in public health and politics (Schneider et al., 1993), respondents allocated responsibility for prevention efforts to both the federal government and to individuals. Less responsibility was given to state and local governments. The federal government was assigned major responsibility for improving health in the areas of AIDS/HIV, maternal and infant health, and the detection and control of major chronic diseases such as hypertension, heart disease, cancer and diabetes. Black leaders may have limited faith in the prospects for adequate funding for state and local agencies to address these issues (Schneider et al., 1993).

However, some statewide public health programs that are federally sponsored (e.g., by the Centers for Disease Control and Prevention and by the National Cancer Institute) have stipulated the use of community coalitions (with minority representation) for planning and implementing interventions. For example, in an inner-city community in Atlanta, which includes census tracts with public housing projects and low incomes (median family income <$5,000 in the 1990

Census), an intervention aimed at increasing screening rates for breast and cervical cancer among black women was developed primarily by health activists who were members of the Atlanta-based National Black Women's Health Project (Sung et al., 1992; Blumenthal et al., 1995). The interventions were delivered by lay health workers, who were inner-city black women, to the homes of participating black women recruited from community health centers and residents of public and senior citizen housing projects.

It can be argued that the discipline of public health has been a major mechanism not only for improving conditions in blacks communities but also as a catalyst for organizing black communities toward common goals. Many public health programs have included black community groups in the planning, design, and execution of public health projects or interventions aimed at primary and secondary prevention of disease. "Lay public health workers," or residents of predominantly minority communities, often have been used in health education programs and other public health interventions, especially those in inner cities.

Some community health projects in Harlem
While the portrayal of Harlem black men as experiencing the life expectancy of third-world countries (McCord and Freeman, 1990) may have had limited social and political impact, in recent years a number of federal- and/or state-funded public health initiatives have been launched in the Harlem area. A physician- and nurse-assisted smoking cessation program in Harlem (Royce et al., 1995) is one example of the growing movement in public health toward community involvement in public health projects, including strong input by community members, groups, and leaders in planning and implementing such projects.

The Harlem Health Connection was a 3-year project conducted by the American Health Foundation (based in New York City) and funded by the American Cancer Society to develop and test smoking-control interventions targeted to blacks. Other organizations involved in the project were a community health center, a community-based heart project (funded by the New York State Health Department), and Harlem Hospital (Royce et al., 1995).

Data showing large increases (starting around 1987) in assault injuries and other injuries in school-aged children in Central Harlem led to the community-based Safe Kids/Healthy Neighborhoods Injury Prevention Program initiated in 1988 (Davidson et al., 1994; Durkin et al., 1994). The work was funded by the federal government (Centers for Disease Control and Prevention) and by private foundations. Low income has been shown to be a predictor of pediatric injuries, so that high rates in Harlem would be expected in view of the concentration of low income in such a highly segregated area. The Program, involving 26 organizations in its planning and implementation, was followed by a declining incidence rate for injuries among school-aged children in predominantly black Central Harlem.

In addition, the Program developed a series of community improvement programs in Central Harlem to renovate parks and playgrounds, involve children in safe and supervised activities, and provide injury and violence prevention education (along with safety equipment) (Davidson et al., 1994). Residents of inner cities, and especially public housing projects, undoubtedly have lower levels of physical activity due in part to the paucity of safe recreational facilities. Such racial disparities could affect a variety of health-related outcomes including obesity (Chapter 6), chronic diseases, and mental disorders such as mild depression. Community health centers (discussed later) also serve as a catalyst in mobilizing communities to improve the physical environment, such as cleaning up trash, as shown in Boston (Klevens et al., 1992). The challenge for such programs in urban ghettos is obviously formidable.

Black community churches and health centers
Black community churches have become involved in community-based public health interventions. In the Black Church Family Project's survey of 635 churches in the northern United States in 1990–1991, church size and education level of the minister were predictors of the frequency of church-sponsored community health outreach efforts (Thomas et al., 1994). A rural county-wide health promotion program enlisting community leaders was facilitated through "progressive" local black churches, but several problems were identified, including the reluctance of churches to coordinate their efforts with existing community health agencies (Turner et al., 1995). Nevertheless, the role of black churches is an emerging area in community health and health promotion research, consistent with the long tradition of the importance of black churches in black communities and black culture. A strong infrastructure (including churches, civic groups, and block associations) in black communities may not only promote black "political empowerment" but also enhance the "general quality of life," which could affect mortality rates (LaVeist, 1992, 1993).

Community health centers often serve populations that are largely or even predominantly minorities in poor inner-city areas because of residential segregation. Some 150 community health centers were established between 1965 and 1971, and almost 800 additional centers had appeared by 1980 (Sardell, 1988). Among all community and migrant health centers funded in fiscal year 1990, one-third were in urban areas and more than 6 million persons were served with primary and preventive services; 85% of clients had incomes less than 200% of the federal poverty level. Among the 357 (of 538) health centers that responded to a survey, blacks comprised about 25% of the clients (Parham and Stephens, 1992).

Community health centers can be important in reaching low-income blacks, as shown for cancer screening tests. Periodic screening by mammography and clinical breast examinations is widely recognized as important in reducing the risk of death from breast cancer in women aged 50 years and older. A need for more mammography facilities in community health centers has been recognized (Parham and Stevens, 1992). Some community health centers have contracted with mammography facilities at local hospitals or with mammography vans, while others have purchased mammography vans. In Dade County, FL, a coalition of seven primary health-care centers was selected because of accessibility to the "target population" (including poor minority women). Some 9,400 women were screened by a mobile mammography van, and 41% were non-Hispanic blacks (Centers for Disease Control and Prevention, 1991). Among low-income women utilizing county-funded health centers in Long Island who were surveyed in 1988, mammography use in the past year did not vary by race and ethnicity (i.e., 29% in non-Hispanic whites, 29% in non-Hispanic blacks, and 33% in Hispanics), suggesting equity in screening rates (Lane et al., 1992) and the need for increased screening for all racial and ethnic groups.

In some inner-city areas, the density of primary-care physicians may be low. The potential role of community health centers in community-based primary care practices is being recognized in order to improve access of minorities to primary-care physicians, thus improving health status (e.g., by better control of hypertension), and to address the problem of "preventable deaths" (Chapter 6). However, the proportion of the population in need of such services that is actually reached by health centers tends to be low. The movement toward "managed care" involves mainly health maintenance organizations (HMOs), and HMOs have tended not to serve low-income areas. Although competition between health centers and other providers (especially HMOs) for Medicare and Medicaid reimbursement has been a problem historically (Sardell, 1988), "managed care" has been expanded by some state governments to cover the Medicaid population (Freund and Hurley, 1995), and health centers have become part of these new HMOs in some urban areas (e.g., Hartford, CT). There is growing recognition of the need for managed care programs that actually reach the poor, medically underserved minorities with health and social services through coalitions of public hospitals, community health centers, maternal and child health clinics, and community-based minority physicians (Andrulis et al., 1996).

Problems and coalitions
Community-based programs should not be invoked as a panacea for health problems. Not all expensive, large-scale community-based intervention projects have produced measurable changes in outcomes, although recent small-scale interventions in the rural South, involving community coalitions, have apparently improved levels of physical activity and other risk factors for cardiovascular diseases among blacks (Brownson et al., 1996).

In inner cities, attempts to enroll participants in interventions projects encounter obstacles related to the poor quality of life. In Atlanta, problems occurred in recruiting (Sung et al., 1992) and retaining participants in cancer control interventions (Blumenthal et al., 1995). Lack of time to participate in in-home education programs and insufficient interest in cancer control issues may be encountered. Recuitment from multiple settings if often needed in such programs; noteworthy was the success of recruitment by lay public health workers in a cancer control project in public housing projects in Atlanta (Sung et al., 1992).

The movement toward community organization may detract attention from recognition of the potential role of the federal government (Lemann, 1992), although some believe that there has been too much reliance on federal programs by black communities, especially since federal assistance may never materialize (Fuchs, 1990).

Community-based public health interventions may require extensive coalitions of resources to have an impact on the health of the population of an entire city or county. A review of large-scale health intervention studies aimed at reducing cardiovascular diseases and their risk factors concluded that the most effective programs will probably involve integration of "efforts at the community, state and national levels to change both policies and practices" (Carleton et al., 1995). Nationally recognized winners of the Models that Work campaign to improve primary medical care for traditionally underserved populations, sponsored by the Bureau of Primary Healthcare (Health Resources and Services Administration), included a partnership between a community health center in a predominantly black area of Cincinnati, OH, and a university medical center; and a coalition of a health center, a hospital, and a local health department in "one of the nation's poorest communities" (in E. St. Louis, IL) (Hall, 1996). Coalitions involving community health centers, public hospitals, and state and local health departments have addressed inadequate medical treatment of patients with such diseases as hypertension and tuberculosis in inner cities (see next section).

"Directly Observed Therapy" in Inner Cities

An important role for communities may involve the marshalling of resources to meet health policy standards developed at the state or federal level. Public health and medical research has shown the need not only for early identification of persons with medical problems but also for continued follow-up to determine if proper treatment is prescribed and compliance with treatment is continued. Programs in hypertension and tuberculosis have received great attention, especially in large, predominantly minority urban areas.

In 1979, long before "directly observed therapy," a report titled "Estimated Community Impact of Hypertension Control in a High Risk Population" (Ouellet et al., 1979) noted that programs to control hypertension and strokes in Baltimore required continuous surveillance and follow-up to ensure that proper treatment was received by hypertensive patients. However, resources may not be available for uninsured or underinsured persons who use hospital emergency departments for medical care. The role of urban teaching hospitals, where many inner-city blacks receive medical attention (Chapter 6), appears unclear. Medical care at these hospitals (representing about 40% of total hospital beds) is more expensive than at nonteaching hospitals due to the costs of medical education and other factors such as greater use of medical technology. Methods have been developed to estimate the "reimbursement differential" that is warranted for teaching versus nonteaching hospitals (Morey et al., 1995). A greater role for teaching hospitals has been advocated for the medical care of blacks in South Africa (Maxwell, 1995), and a similar recommendation could be made for the United States. The possibility of differential quality of treatment of black and white patients at such hospitals (Chapter 6) requires further study.

Hospitals in inner-city areas have recently begun collaborating in programs aimed at improving the medical follow-up of patients with certain diseases.

In Chicago and New York City, "directly observed therapy" programs, or close follow-up of patients to ensure proper treatment, have been developed in response to federal policy standards of care for tuberculosis, with collaborative efforts among state, county, and municipal health departments. A special issue of the *Journal of Public Health Management and Practice* (Vol. 1, No. 4, Fall 1995) was devoted to collaborative programs in directly observed therapy for tuberculosis and HIV. One example involved Harlem Hospital and the New York State Department of Health.

McCord and Freeman (1990) noted that tuberculosis patients were often lost to follow-up at Harlem Hospital. Loss to follow-up and problems of compliance with therapeutic regimens are common in high-poverty, segregated areas because of lack of proper medical care, multiple social problems (including homelessness), and lack of social support. After a period of rapidly increasing rates of newly diagnosed tuberculosis in New York City (especially after 1983) (Wallace, 1994), efforts to improve follow-up and compliance, along with other public health measures, were associated with a decline in the case rate for tuberculosis (Frankel, 1994, 1995).

Lack of proper medical follow-up in New York City has also contributed to the rise of tuberculosis patients who rapidly become resistant to certain antituberculosis drugs (such as fluoroquinolone). Improper care resulted in treatment with only one drug (monotherapy), whereas multidrug regimens are needed for proper care. Poor adherence and "selective drug taking" by patients lost to medical observation were involved (Sullivan et al., 1995). Prevention of the emergence and transmission of drug-resistant tuberculosis requires proper follow-up and medical care, which presents difficulties for patients living in high-poverty areas.

With regard to the epidemiology of discrimination and racism, the example of tuberculosis also shows that there may be a double standard in the definition of public health problems or "epidemics." That is, "high" rates of disease or death in predominantly minority areas may be acceptable (or deemed incorrigible) until other areas (not occupied mainly by minorities) are affected. It was widely assumed that tuberculosis had been controlled in the United States in 1980, despite rates of 50 per 100,000 in Central Harlem. However, in 1991 widespread concern about tuberculosis emerged when the case rate for all of New York City reached 50 per 100,000. By 1991, the rate in Central Harlem had increased to 221 per 100,000 (Frieden, 1994). If public health officials had been as alarmed about Central Harlem in 1980 as they were about all of New York in 1991, "much of the city's epidemic might have been avoided" (Frieden, 1994). Central Harlem and Lower East Side areas were the primary "epicenters" of tuberculosis around 1979 (with about 50 cases per square mile), when housing overcrowding was "at a more manageable level" than in 1990 (Wallace, 1994). Overcrowding has long been known to be a major factor in the spread of tuberculosis (as mentioned in Chapter 6).

Thus, in addition to the overrepresentation of blacks in a secondary (low-status) dual labor market, and the persistence of a dual housing market involved in de facto segregation (Chapter 2), there may be a dual standard in the definition of public health problems. However, it is unclear if the failure to recognize an epidemic of tuberculosis in Harlem in 1979 was due to a lack of concern about Harlem or to the fact that the high case rate was limited to one area (whatever its racial and ethnic composition).

The prospects for expanded funding in the mid-1990s are in question for "directly observed therapy (treatment)." In 1995, the political movement was toward block grants that would allow the states to make decisions about allocating funds for "directly observed treatment" of tuberculosis, despite successes in controlling tuberculosis in New York and New Jersey. The loss of funds specifically targeting such intensive follow-up of patients, which is expensive, would probably wipe out the gains made in control of tuberculosis in urban areas (Centers for Disease Control and Prevention, 1995; Reichman, 1996).

The need for community-based health outreach workers in such therapy programs also has been recognized, along with the impact of various social problems, such as homelessness (Chapter 3) and drug and alcohol abuse, on compliance with therapy. Empirical studies and (especially) intervention projects in "directly observed therapy" will not be "simple or cheap" (Bayer and Wilkinson, 1995). The potential role of voluntary community organizations (including churches), discussed earlier, should be considered. The challenge is formidable, if one considers the multiple public health problems that could benefit from intensive monitoring and follow-up of poor minority patients for compliance with treatment. Other conditions potentially amenable to "directly observed therapy" programs include asthma, smoking cessation, and alcohol and drug abuse treatment.

Segregation, Health, and American Values

Despite all the efforts to improve medical care and public health, there are limits to all such programs. They may be viewed as interim and partial solutions to problems that reflect deeper social ills. Higher rates of death among blacks in more segregated urban areas are symptomatic of poorer quality of life, environment, and medical care. The decade following the civil rights movement provides the clearest evidence of social progress for blacks in terms of trends in poverty rates, education, and mortality rates (Cooper, 1993; West, 1994). However, time trends in black social class and segregation (Chapters 2 and 3), along with black mortality rates in hypersegregated urban areas (Chapter 5), reinforce the view in *A Common Destiny: Blacks and American Society* that "time alone [will] not resolve America's racial problems" (Jaynes and Williams, 1989).

In his 1944 State of the Union address, President Roosevelt called "freedom from want" as a "second Bill of Rights" that included not only rights to a "useful and remunerative job" that provides income for adequate food, clothing, and recreation but also "the right to adequate medical care" (Leuchtenberg, 1963). The Roosevelt Administration, however, avoided civil rights issues (including the desegregation of the military) in order to maintain Congressional support for other programs. Roosevelt's speech was made just as Myrdal's *An American Dilemma* was received by reviewers (Jackson, 1990). Part of Myrdal's "American creed" ideal was that while economic inequality was not wrong, "no population group" should be "allowed to fall under a certain minimum standard of living" and blacks "should be awarded equal opportunities" (Jackson, 1990). The early part of the Great Depression has been characterized as a period of transient expansion of "community-oriented values" which was gradually replaced by the economic boom associated with World War II and the New Deal's emphasis on high consumption. In the *Lancet* editorial "Against the Culture of Contentment" (Anon. 1993), the contrast between the numbers of physicians in Manhattan (3.3 per 1,000 people) and in the Bronx (0.2 per 1000), inhabited predominantly by minorities, was cited as one example of gross inequities that are accepted by society.

A *Lancet* "viewpoint" article went so far as to pose the question of whether "inequality" was actually "bad for the national health" (Charlton, 1994). Because there may be an absence of a threshold at which health benefits from increasing income cease, the "profound" policy consequences were that "redistribution of resources" was not a desirable option for improving the health of a nation. Some of the "commodity" of health would be transferred "from the rich to the poor." Similar arguments have been advanced in the debate about universal health insurance, where the security of those able to afford extensive, high-technology medical care could be threatened. These arguments dismiss the moral issue of raising the standard of living and health for the poor to a basic minimum level.

With regard to health care reform, it seems debatable that there is "good agreement" with the concept (Eddy, 1991) that some people can receive a very high level of medical care (at their own expense) provided that the lowest level of care "covers everything that is essential." However, this concept is consistent with "value-based" ideas that health care access is a basic "right" for all Americans (Dougherty, 1988; Jencks, 1993). "Federalization" of Medicaid has been proposed, with a national reimbursement formula that takes into account local variation in costs of living and health care in order to produce the "moral benefit" of a national standard for a "decent minimum level of health care that no American would have to go without" (Dougherty, 1988).

If the American ethos of individual responsibility influences the debate about health insurance reform, proposals offer alternatives to such direct federal interference. Individuals could be required to obtain minimal adequate coverage that would be subsidized for low-income persons through federal tax credits and other adjustment (Pauly et al., 1992). A voucher system, which would allow individual choice of health care plans, could also be used.

As mentioned earlier, health care reform will not solve more basic social problems, such as those affecting quality of life in inner cities. A "value-based" approach to health care reform by "social solidarity," acknowledged to be "rarely mentioned in discussions of U.S. health policy," was compared with the U.S. public education system (Priester, 1992). De facto segregation in public schools was not mentioned. However, the "values" argument of Priester could easily be extended to other social and health problems involving glaring inequities, including high poverty rates among children and in ghettos.

If "value-based" approaches are rejected, "self interest" approaches to helping the poor blacks in ghettos must be presented as somehow beneficial to nonblacks and nonpoor. In a "culture of contentment" (Galbraith, 1992) guarded by the majority, arguments could be based on fears of periodic urban riots (as warned by Myrdal) (Chapter 3), the mounting costs of crime and incarceration, and other chronic costs of maintaining ghettos. An underlying hypothesis would be that ghetto violence is very strongly related to the social and economic conditions of ghettos ("concentration" or "neighborhood" effects) (Chapter 4). Economists might compare the economic costs of the persistence of ghettos with the costs of removing ghettos or of replacing the system of low-income housing projects with a legally mandated (and enforced) voucher system with designated residences located outside ghettos. Some partial answers may have been obtained, as various states have estimated the effects of violence (trauma patients) in urban communities on total "uncompensated" health care costs. These costs divert funds from the limited health care pools of urban hospitals and detract from primary care for other diseases (such as hypertension) common in blacks (Fong, 1995).

Meanwhile, "value-based" approaches to problems in inner cities are being addressed by black communities. While there is increasing interest in "black community" power structures and solidarity, a potential drawback is that the "two nations" will grow farther apart. Also, there are obvious limits to the success of programs promoting community "self-determination" in a national (and increasingly international) economy. A similar dilemma was confronted long ago by W.E.B. Du Bois, who did not reject integration as a long-term goal while advocating a process of increasing "economic power, political unity, and self-respect" (Jackson, 1990) in black communities faced by persistent segregation. The development of black political factions in mayoral electoral campaigns and the limited impact of increases in both black voter participation and the number of black mayors on quality of life for urban blacks (Peterson, 1994) underscore the complexities.

Problems such as inner-city violence and out-of-wedlock births also must be addressed by black communities (Joint Center for Political Studies, 1983), along with increasing the self-esteem of ghetto residents (both men and women) often removed from the mainstream workforce (Wilson, 1987, 1991a,b). Acceptance of the role of moral leadership in black communities (since the time of W.E.B. Du Bois), however, should not preclude the development of coalition efforts that involve federal, state, and local governments in addressing a variety of problems such as those related to public health in metropolitan areas.

Fuchs (1993) proposed that the President of the United States give a speech presenting a "policy agenda" that includes stronger enforcement of antidiscriminatory legislation. The goal would be to reduce housing discrimination as part of a "plan to end the segregation that has been imposed on African-Americans . . . and dark-skinned Americans in our inner cities." How to find resources for such programs as vouchers for housing outside the ghettos, Gatreaux-like projects (Chapter 3), jobs and child care for "welfare" mothers, and expansion of Head Start and Healthy Start is an important question. As mentioned earlier, in addition to federal enforcement of civil rights laws, educational programs aimed at reducing resistance to segregation also would be needed as part of such a "policy agenda."

Movement of more blacks out of ghettos would further dramatize the problem of decaying inner cities. In *The New American Ghetto*, sociologist-photojournalist C.J. Vergara (1995) has proposed minimal preservation or stabilization of certain architecturally interesting, abandoned buildings of the ghettos as "ruins" in "national parks" rather than destroying all of the edifices and replacing them with poorly constructed buildings. In Vergara's words (1995), "While they last, we have our ruins" to remind us about "our abject failure to create a just society," yet begging us "to come home and perhaps try again."

A *Lancet* editorial on inequality of health by social class, racial and ethnic group and age advocated the selection of "achievable" aims or goals from the "torrent of problems" and the marshalling of political resources by creating a sense of urgency (Anon. 1995b). In addition, the need for a "champion" of such causes was acknowledged. The abolition of slavery (in Britain) was mentioned as one example of an achieved goal that had desirable effects on inequalities in health and other aspects of life despite the failure to "halt racial discrimination." Perhaps the power of the message for the causes of reducing urban segregation and improving the quality of life for those left behind in the ghettos could be increased by the use of statistics on mortality of African-American infants and young adults in Harlem (McCord and Freeman, 1990) and in other hypersegregated metropolitan areas (as compiled in this book).

The findings on overall mortality rates for young adult black men (Chapter 5) confirm McCord and Freeman's suspicion (1990) that high death rates hold for black adults in other hypersegregated cities. McCord and Freeman's analysis (1990) of cause-specific mortality in one hypersegregated area (Harlem) should be updated, and similar analyses should be conducted in other hypersegregated areas. Preferably, local public health departments should be involved in such studies in order to facilitate the planning of interventions. Infant mortality trends, a "social mirror" or sensitive indicator of social progress (Wise and Pursley, 1992; Yankauer, 1990), indicate a persisting (or recently expanding) black–white gap that deserves special attention in social and health policies. The persistence of high black infant mortality rates (greater than 20 per 1,000 black live births) in highly segregated metropolitan areas (Chapter 5) accentuate this need.

Mortality statistics add objective support to the portraits of despair facing a "young black generation . . . up against the forces of death, destruction, and disease unprecedented in the everyday life of black urban people" (West, 1994). At the very least, these statistics may promote the epidemiologic study of the consequences of American apartheid for African Americans.

Appendix

Some of the tables in this Appendix provide the results of multiple regression models. Multiple linear regression analysis involves the development of models that use independent variables that may be associated with the dependent variable of interest; such as mortality rates by MSA or PMSA. If the association (measured by the correlation coefficient, or Pearson r) between two independent variables is too strong (e.g., 0.90 or greater), then the problem of "multi-colinearity" must be addressed, usually by excluding one of the two intercorrelated variables. The independent variables are included in a model in which the association between each independent variable and the dependent variables is adjusted for the (linear) effects of the other independent variable(s) in the model. If certain statistical assumptions are met, a statistical test (based on the Gaussian or normal distribution) can be applied to each regression coefficient. This tests the "null" hypothesis that the coefficient is zero, or that the independent variable has no association with the dependent variable, when other independent variables are included in the model.

The results of the analysis usually include estimates of the regression coefficients for each independent variable, the t value or ratio of the regression coefficient to its standard error, and an intercept value or constant for the equation. R^2 (R squared) is a measure of how well the model "fits" the data, and the proportion of variation in the dependent variable that is "explained" by the model. The R^2 values in the tables are "adjusted" or more conservative measures of goodness of fit of the model. Some computer "packages" commonly used for multiple linear regression analysis are summarized by Afifi and Clark (1984).

Table A-1. Black (B) and white (W) infant mortality rates (per 1,000 live births) in 92 metropolitan areas in 1989–1991

Area*	Infant mortality rate			Poverty rate ratio B/W	Segregation index
	Black	White	Ratio B/W		
Akron, OH, PMSA	18.3	7.5	2.43	3.60	74
Albany, GA, MSA	21.6	7.8	2.76	5.48	70
Atlanta, GA, MSA	17.4	7.6	2.30	4.15	73
Atlantic City, NJ, MSA	23.8	7.2	3.29	3.20	72
Augusta, GA–SC, MSA	16.6	9.7	1.70	3.53	56
Austin, TX, MSA	12.8	5.6	2.28	2.22	57
Baltimore, MD, MSA	15.7	6.8	2.31	4.30	75
Baton Rouge, LA, MSA	17.6	6.7	2.63	4.00	73
Beaumont–Port Arthur, TX, MSA	18.0	6.9	2.59	3.54	76
Birmingham, AL, MSA	18.1	7.0	2.59	3.41	79
Boston–Lawrence–Salem–Lowell–Brockton, MA, NECMA	12.6	6.3	1.99	3.44	70
Bridgeport–Stamford–Norwalk–Danbury, CT, NECMA	17.4	5.6	3.12	3.48	69
Buffalo, NY, PMSA	19.6	7.3	2.69	4.56	84
Charleston, SC, MSA	18.4	7.1	2.58	4.20	58
Charlotte–Gastonia–Rock Hill, NC–SC, MSA	17.8	7.5	2.37	3.69	65
Chattanooga, TN–GA, MSA	12.8	9.5	1.34	2.90	78
Chicago, IL, PMSA	24.5	8.4	2.94	5.17	87
Cincinnati, OH–KY–IN, PMSA	17.2	7.5	2.30	4.25	80
Cleveland, OH, PMSA	20.9	8.2	2.55	4.56	86
Columbia, SC, MSA	13.9	8.6	1.62	3.28	63
Columbus, GA–AL, MSA	17.2	9.4	1.83	3.38	62
Columbus, OH, MSA	17.7	8.5	2.08	3.11	71
Dallas, TX, PMSA	16.0	7.5	2.12	3.71	66
Dayton–Springfield, OH, MSA	16.2	7.3	2.23	3.42	78
Denver, CO, PMSA	18.0	8.0	2.24	3.28	66
Detroit, MI, PMSA	22.4	7.3	3.07	4.65	89
Fayetteville–Springdale, AR, MSA	16.9	8.1	2.10	3.15	41
Flint, MI, MSA	21.5	9.1	2.37	3.29	84
Fort Lauderdale–Hollywood–Pompano Beach, FL, PMSA	19.5	6.5	2.98	3.83	73
Gary–Hammond, IN, PMSA	16.0	8.5	1.88	4.89	91
Grand Rapids, MI, MSA	19.2	7.8	2.47	4.91	74
Greensboro–Winston-Salem–High Point, NC, MSA	18.9	8.3	2.27	3.07	68
Greenville–Spartansburg, SC, MSA	16.4	9.7	1.69	3.06	63
Hartford–New Britain–Middletown, CT, NECMA	18.4	7.2	2.57	4.95	71
Houston, TX, PMSA	16.0	6.8	2.36	2.97	69
Indianapolis, IN, MSA	20.6	8.6	2.40	3.80	80
Jackson, MS, MSA	13.9	8.1	1.72	5.34	75
Jacksonville, FL, MSA	16.2	8.0	2.03	3.95	65
Jersey City, NJ, PMSA	15.5	8.4	1.83	2.07	70
Kansas City, MO–KS, MSA	17.7	7.3	2.44	4.07	76
Killeen–Temple, TX, MSA	13.7	8.2	1.67	1.94	45
Lakeland–Winter Haven, FL, MSA	17.1	8.8	1.93	3.20	72
Las Vegas, NV, MSA	18.0	7.5	2.40	2.83	51
Little Rock–North Little Rock, AR, MSA	14.3	8.6	1.66	3.35	68
Los Angeles–Long Beach, CA, PMSA	18.0	7.4	2.45	2.00	71
Louisville, KY–IN, MSA	16.6	8.3	2.01	3.56	74

(continued)

Table A-1. (Continued)

Area*	Infant mortality rate			Poverty rate ratio B/W	Segregation index
	Black	White	Ratio B/W		
Macon–Warner Robins, GA, MSA	22.4	7.7	2.92	4.49	60
Memphis, TN–AR–MS, MSA	19.9	7.6	2.61	5.21	76
Miami–Hialeah, FL, PMSA	15.1	6.4	2.38	2.13	75
Milwaukee, WI, PMSA	16.2	7.2	2.27	7.12	84
Minneapolis–St Paul, MN, MSA	22.8	6.5	3.52	6.27	65
Mobile, AL, MSA	15.1	8.1	1.86	3.97	74
Monroe, LA, MSA	15.9	11.0	1.45	4.40	76
Montgomery, AL, MSA	17.7	9.3	1.92	5.14	67
Nashville, TN, MSA	17.1	8.9	1.91	3.24	66
Nassau–Suffolk, NY, PMSA	23.2	6.5	3.56	3.49	79
New Haven–Waterbury–Meriden, CT, NECMA	17.1	6.7	2.54	4.76	70
New Orleans, LA, MSA	16.2	7.9	2.05	4.04	74
New York, NY, PMSA	17.6	8.9	1.97	2.30	78
Newark, NJ, PMSA	18.8	6.2	3.02	4.33	83
Norfolk–Virginia Beach–Newport News, VA, MSA	21.2	9.6	2.21	4.25	57
Oklahoma City, OK, MSA	16.5	9.7	1.71	2.85	65
Omaha, NE–IA, MSA	17.2	6.6	2.60	3.62	72
Orlando, FL, MSA	15.3	6.3	2.44	3.62	65
Pensacola, FL, MSA	16.7	7.7	2.17	3.46	63
Philadelphia, PA–NJ, PMSA	20.6	7.1	2.89	4.55	82
Phoenix, AZ, MSA	19.3	8.3	2.33	2.88	51
Pittsburgh, PA, PMSA	24.1	7.5	3.24	3.59	75
Providence–Pawtucket–Woonsocket, RI, NECMA	16.5	8.2	2.02	3.08	69
Raleigh–Durham, NC, MSA	19.2	6.5	2.97	3.15	57
Richmond–Petersburg, VA, MSA	18.7	7.0	2.67	4.22	64
Riverside–San Bernardino, CA, PMSA	19.8	8.6	2.29	2.10	49
Rochester, NY, MSA	20.7	6.4	3.24	5.46	70
Sacramento, CA, MSA	17.9	7.5	2.39	2.67	58
St Louis, MO–IL, MSA	19.1	6.8	2.80	4.97	81
San Antonio, TX, MSA	14.4	10.3	1.40	1.63	57
San Diego, CA, MSA	16.9	6.9	2.45	2.54	59
San Francisco, CA, PMSA	14.8	6.3	2.36	3.46	65
San Jose, CA, PMSA	18.0	6.5	2.78	2.40	45
Savannah, GA, MSA	17.9	9.4	1.90	4.39	71
Seattle, WA, PMSA	19.8	6.6	3.03	3.56	60
Shreveport, LA, MSA	15.7	6.3	2.48	4.93	67
Syracuse, NY, MSA	20.1	9.3	2.17	4.19	76
Tallahassee, FL, MSA	15.3	6.8	2.24	2.75	59
Tampa–St. Petersburg–Clearwater, FL, MSA	18.7	8.0	2.34	3.68	74
Toledo, OH, MSA	16.2	8.7	1.87	3.74	77
Trenton, NJ, PMSA	21.7	7.7	2.81	4.90	76
Tulsa, OK, MSA	15.2	8.1	1.87	3.50	69
Washington, DC–MD–VA, MSA	20.1	6.8	2.95	3.50	68
West Palm Beach–Boca Raton–Delray Beach, FL, MSA	16.9	8.3	2.03	4.89	78
Wilmington, DE-NJ-MD, PMSA	21.4	8.5	2.52	3.91	64
Youngstown–Warren, OH, MSA	20.3	8.5	2.39	3.97	79

*MSA, Metropolitan Statistical Area; PMSA, Primary Metropolitan Statistical Area; NECMA, New England County Metropolitan Area.

Table A-2. Prediction of the average annual infant mortality rate in blacks and whites in 92 U.S. MSAs in 1989–1991 by multiple regression*

Independent variable	Dependent variable					
	Black mortality rate			White mortality rate		
	Coefficient	t	p	Coefficient	t	p
Race-specific poverty in 1989	−0.062	−1.63	0.107	0.177	3.91	<0.001
Segregation index, 1990	+0.075	2.64	0.010	0.040	0.41	0.685
Constant		14.498			6.020	
Adjusted R^2		0.058			0.128	

*t, The regression coefficient divided by its standard error. The segregation index is the index of dissimilarity (see Chapter 2 for formula) multiplied by 100 (as reported by Farley and Frey, 1992, 1994).

Table A-3. Characteristics of 34 MSAs used in analyses of infant mortality rate (IMR) and quality of neighborhood or housing for blacks

				Occupied housing units with black householder		
MSA	Black IMR	Black poverty	Segregation index	1.01+ PPR*	Lower quality neighborhood	Lower quality housing
Atlanta	17.42	22	73	0.03	0.10	0.05
Baltimore	15.71	23	75	0.03	0.15	0.06
Birmingham	18.05	31	79	0.06	0.10	0.05
Boston	12.59	22	70	0.05	0.15	0.08
Buffalo	19.56	37	84	0.01	0.10	0.03
Chicago	24.52†	30	87	0.06	0.21	0.07
Cincinnati	17.21	34	80	0.03	0.16	0.08
Cleveland	20.92†	31	86	0.03	0.13	0.05
Columbus	17.73	29	71	0.02	0.15	0.06
Dallas	15.96	27	66	0.07	0.13	0.06
Denver	17.95	25	66	0.01	0.13	0.05
Detroit	22.43†	33	89	0.02	0.17	0.07
Houston	16.04	28	69	0.05	0.13	0.06
Indianapolis	20.62†	26	80	0.05	0.13	0.09
Kansas City	17.73	28	76	0.05	0.14	0.08
Los Angeles	18.03	21	71	0.05	0.15	0.06
Memphis	19.86	35	76	0.08	0.11	0.07
Miami	15.09	30	75	0.09	0.11	0.07
Milwaukee	16.24	41	84	0.05	0.20	0.10
Minneapolis	22.75†	37	65	0.06	0.22	0.09
New Orleans	16.19	41	74	0.07	0.13	0.05
New York, NY	17.59	25	78	0.09	0.18	0.08
Norfolk	21.16†	25	57	0.03	0.08	0.06
Philadelphia	20.60	26	82	0.04	0.17	0.04
Phoenix	19.32	27	51	0.07	0.11	0.07
Pittsburgh	24.14†	36	75	0.03	0.19	0.07
Riverside	19.76	20	49	0.07	0.10	0.04
St. Louis	19.13	31	81	0.06	0.15	0.06
San Antonio	14.41	26	57	0.03	0.11	0.07
San Diego	16.85	21	59	0.07	0.13	0.06
San Jose	18.04	13	45	0.01	0.09	0.05
Seattle	19.84	22	60	0.03	0.06	0.04
Tampa	18.66	33	74	0.06	0.11	0.07
Washington	20.13†	13	68	0.02	0.11	0.05

*PPR, Persons per room.
† Black infant mortality rate >20 per 1,000 per year (average annual rate for 1989–1991). For full titles of MSAs, see Table A-1.

Table A-4. Prediction of black/white mortality ratio for men and women in 38 MSAs for ages 15–24, 25–34, and 35–44 years, 1982–1986

Age (years)	Univariate model		Bivariate model		
	Black/white poverty ratio B	Model R^2	Black/white poverty ratio B	Segregation index B	Model R^2
MEN					
15–24	0.124*	0.117	0.035	1.618*	0.232
25–34	0.443†	0.466	0.292*	2.742†	0.569
35–44	0.370‡	0.399	0.277†	1.686	0.446
15–44	0.324‡	0.406	0.206†	2.139*	0.508
WOMEN					
15–24	0.072	0.058	0.022	0.913	0.111
25–34	0.193*	0.124	0.079	2.068	0.161
35–44	0.228‡	0.336	0.146*	1.472*	0.418
15–44	0.179‡	0.282	0.085	1.511*	0.399

From Polednak (1993).

The rate for 15–44 year olds is an age-adjusted rate. The black/white ratio of poverty rate (in the 1980 Census) was coded to two decimal places; segregation index, three decimal places (from Massey and Denton, 1987). B is the regression coefficient (see text).

*p < 0.05

†p < 0.01

‡p < 0.001 for t-test on regression coefficient (see text).

Table A-5. Names and characteristics of 50 MSAs used in analyses of death rates in young adults, 1990–1991

Area*	Segregation index	Black poverty (%)	White poverty (%)	Black/white poverty ratio
MSAs WITH >1 MILLION TOTAL POPULATION IN 1980				
Anaheim–SantaAna, CA, PMSA	43	9.7	6.7	1.45
Atlanta, GA, MSA	73	22.4	5.4	4.15
Baltimore, MD, MSA	75	23.2	5.4	4.30
Boston–Lawrence–Lowell–Brockton, MA, NECMA	70	21.7	6.3	3.44
Buffalo, NY, PMSA	84	37.4	8.2	4.56
Chicago, IL, PMSA	87	30.0	5.8	5.17
Cincinnati, OH–KY–IN, PMSA	80	34.0	8.0	4.25
Cleveland, OH, PMSA	86	31.0	6.8	4.56
Columbus, OH, MSA	71	28.9	9.3	3.11
Dallas, TX, PMSA	66	26.7	7.2	3.71
Denver, CO, PMSA	66	24.6	7.5	3.28
Detroit, MI, PMSA	89	33.0	7.1	4.65
Fort Lauderdale–Hollywood–Pampano Beach, FL, PMSA	73	26.8	7.0	3.83
Houston, TX, PMSA	69	27.9	9.4	2.97
Indianapolis, IN, MSA	80	26.2	6.9	3.80
Kansas City, MO–KS, MSA	76	28.1	6.9	4.07
Los Angeles–Long Beach, CA, PMSA	71	21.2	10.6	2.00
Miami–Hialeah, FL, PMSA	75	30.3	14.2	2.13
Milwaukee, WI, PMSA	84	41.3	5.8	7.12
Minneapolis–St. Paul, MN–WI, MSA	65	37.0	5.9	6.27
Nassau–Suffolk, NY, PMSA	79	12.2	3.5	3.49
New Orleans, LA, MSA	74	40.8	10.1	4.04
New York, NY, PMSA	78	24.8	10.8	2.30
Newark, NJ, PMSA	83	19.9	4.6	4.33
Philadelphia, PA–NJ, PMSA	82	25.5	5.6	4.55
Phoenix, AZ, MSA	51	27.4	9.5	2.88
Pittsburgh, PA, PMSA	75	35.9	10.0	3.59
Portland, OR, PMSA	68	29.3	8.7	3.37
Riverside–San Bernardino, CA, PMSA	49	20.4	9.7	2.10
Sacramento, CA, MSA	58	24.0	9.0	2.67
St. Louis, MO–IL, MSA	81	31.3	6.3	4.97
San Antonio, TX, MSA	57	26.4	16.2	1.63
San Diego, CA, MSA	59	21.3	8.4	2.54
San Jose, CA, PMSA	46	12.7	5.3	2.40
Seattle, WA, PMSA	60	21.7	6.1	3.56
Tampa–St. Petersburg–Clearwater, FL, MSA	74	33.1	9.0	3.68
Washington, DC–MD–VA, MSA	68	12.6	3.6	3.50
MSAs WITH >150,000 BLACKS IN 1990				
Baton Rouge, LA, MSA	73	39.6	9.9	4.00
Birmingham, AL, MSA	79	31.4	9.2	3.41
Charleston, SC, MSA	58	31.9	7.6	4.20
Charlotte–Gastonia–RockHill, NC–SC, MSA	65	22.9	6.2	3.69
Greensboro–Winston-Salem–High Point, NC, MSA	68	21.8	7.1	3.07
Jackson, MS, MSA	75	36.3	6.8	5.34
Jacksonville, FL, MSA	65	29.2	7.4	3.95
Memphis, TN–AR–MS, MSA	76	34.9	6.7	5.21

(continued)

Table A-5. Names and characteristics of 50 MSAs used in analyses of death rates in young adults, 1990–1991 (Continued)

Area*	Segregation index	Black poverty (%)	White poverty (%)	Black/white poverty ratio
Nashville, TN, MSA	66	27.2	8.4	3.24
Norfolk–Virginia Beach–Newport News, VA, MSA	57	25.1	5.9	4.25
Oakland, CA, PMSA	69	21.1	5.9	3.58
Raleigh–Durham, NC, MSA	57	20.5	6.5	3.15
Richmond–Petersburg, VA, MSA	64	21.1	5.0	4.22

*MSA, Metropolitan Statistical Area; PMSA, Primary Metropolitan Statistical Area; NECMA, New England County Metropolitan Area.

Table A-6. Multiple regression analysis of black (B) mortality rate and black/white (B/W) ratio of mortality rates in males 15–24 to 35–44 years old in 50 MSAs, 1990–1991*

	Black mortality rate				B/W mortality ratio		
Variable	Coefficient	t	p	Variable	Coefficient	t	p
AGES 15–24 YEARS							
Poverty, black	0.041	0.68	0.503	B/W poverty	0.247	2.48	0.006
Segregation	0.858	2.10	0.041	Segregation	0.018	2.03	0.048
Constant	18.447			Constant	0.047		
Adjusted R²	0.114			Adjusted R²	0.351		
AGEs 25–34 YEARS							
Poverty, black	−0.038	−0.49	0.630	B/W poverty	0.358	3.87	<0.001
Segregation	2.995	5.67	<0.001	Segregation	0.030	3.13	0.001
Constant	−45.068			Constant	−0.986		
Adjusted R²	0.432			Adjusted R²	0.533		
AGES 35–44 YEARS							
Poverty, black	−1.046	−2.83	0.028	B/W poverty	0.258	2.28	0.027
Segregation	16.266	6.52	<0.001	Segregation	0.032	2.81	0.007
Constant	−182.673			Constant	−0.764		
Adjusted R²	0.453			Adjusted R²	0.370		
AGE-STANDARDIZED RATE, AGES 15–44 YEARS							
Poverty, black	−0.330	−1.57	0.122	B/W poverty	0.292	3.38	0.002
Segregation	9.030	6.38	<0.001	Segregation	0.029	3.28	0.002
Constant	−84.757			Constant	−0.722		
Adjusted R²	0.462			Adjusted R²	0.543		

*The segregation indexes were coded as 43–89. Poverty rates were coded to three decimal places (e.g., 0.200 for 20.0% poverty rate).

Table A-7. Multiple regression analysis of black (B) and black/white ratios of age-adjusted mortality rate for females (15–44 years old) in 50 MSAs, 1990–1991

Variable	Black death rate			Black/white death rate ratio		
	Coefficient	t	p	Coefficient	t	p
Poverty*	−0.115	−1.42	0.162	0.003	0.04	0.969
Segregation	2.659	4.85	<0.001	0.029	3.26	0.002
Constant	12.903			0.091		
Adjusted R²	0.317			0.223		

*"Poverty" is black poverty rate for prediction of black death rate, and black/white ratio of poverty rates for prediction of black/white death rate ratio.

Table A-8. Black/white ratios of mortality rates for young adult males and age-adjusted mortality rates (ages 15–44 years) in 50 MSAs, 1990–1991

MSA	Black/white ratios of age-specific rates			Age-adjusted rates		
	15–24	25–34	35–44	Black	White	Ratio
MSAs WITH >1 MILLION TOTAL POPULATION IN 1980						
Anaheim	1.05	0.49	1.10	195.6	245.0	0.80
Atlanta	2.23	2.62	2.82	543.1	206.0	2.64
Baltimore	2.21	4.01	4.09	593.0	160.8	3.69
Boston	3.05	2.07	2.05	472.5	213.0	2.22
Buffalo	2.72	2.97	3.43	440.7	139.2	3.17
Chicago	2.81	3.65	3.28	656.9	199.1	3.30
Cincinnati	1.91	1.91	2.00	289.0	148.0	1.95
Cleveland	2.86	3.30	2.97	488.9	160.1	3.05
Columbus	2.96	1.99	1.80	339.9	162.1	2.10
Dallas	2.26	1.72	1.80	473.5	252.1	1.88
Denver	1.23	1.51	1.35	297.2	216.0	1.38
Detroit	3.68	3.59	3.86	600.8	161.1	3.73
Fort Lauderdale	2.35	1.89	1.80	456.0	239.1	1.91
Houston	1.45	1.64	1.64	511.1	320.0	1.60
Indianapolis	1.63	1.96	2.38	389.9	188.9	2.06
Kansas City	2.40	2.65	2.13	438.9	185.2	2.37
Los Angeles	1.47	1.58	1.61	566.8	362.0	1.57
Miami	2.63	2.23	1.97	604.9	281.4	2.15
Milwaukee	3.55	3.63	2.85	472.7	144.9	3.26
Minneapolis	2.74	2.78	2.49	354.9	134.8	2.63
Nassau-Suffolk	2.44	3.25	3.64	542.6	164.4	3.30
New Orleans	2.77	2.85	2.01	636.6	259.7	2.45
New York, NY	1.69	1.59	1.72	746.6	446.8	1.67
Newark	2.57	4.28	5.61	772.3	166.4	4.64
Philadelphia	2.64	2.85	3.03	524.1	181.3	2.89
Phoenix	1.42	1.23	1.65	329.1	226.2	1.45
Pittsburgh	1.88	3.35	2.77	431.8	155.0	2.79
Portland	2.50	2.56	1.85	420.3	188.4	2.23
Riverside	1.32	1.43	1.18	188.8	145.3	1.30

(continued)

Table A-8. Black/white ratios of mortality rates for young adult males and age-adjusted mortality rates (ages 15–44 years) in 50 MSAs, 1990–1991 (Continued)

MSA	Black/white ratios of age-specific rates			Age-adjusted rates		
	15–24	25–34	35–44	Black	White	Ratio
Sacramento	1.78	1.24	1.74	369.7	235.5	1.57
St. Louis	3.15	3.74	3.63	590.2	166.1	3.55
San Antonio	1.78	1.29	1.04	383.7	296.2	1.30
San Diego	1.14	0.97	1.35	282.3	238.5	1.18
San Jose	1.57	0.93	1.40	223.0	174.2	1.28
Seattle	2.41	2.12	1.98	380.5	179.8	2.12
Tampa	1.71	2.19	1.80	433.2	226.7	1.91
Washington, DC	3.64	3.23	3.29	513.5	153.5	3.35
MSAs WITH >150,000 BLACKS IN 1990						
Baton Rouge	1.66	2.37	2.82	525.8	220.2	2.39
Birmingham	2.00	2.33	2.99	536.0	215.3	2.49
Charleston	1.94	2.88	2.44	440.2	177.6	2.48
Charlotte	1.84	3.07	3.65	524.5	174.6	3.00
Greensboro	1.22	2.86	3.20	412.6	161.2	2.56
Jackson, MS	1.38	2.06	2.32	404.0	204.3	1.98
Jacksonville	2.91	2.85	2.63	559.7	203.2	2.75
Memphis	2.53	2.27	2.85	457.0	177.9	2.57
Nashville	1.78	1.89	2.22	386.8	193.3	2.00
Norfolk	2.27	3.02	2.55	364.2	136.1	2.66
Oakland	2.96	2.56	2.46	550.2	211.7	2.60
Raleigh	1.97	2.49	3.21	365.3	135.0	2.71
Richmond	2.62	2.62	2.52	424.5	164.8	2.58

Table A-9. Black/white ratios of mortality rates for young adult females and age-adjusted mortality rates (ages 15–44 years) in 50 MSAs, 1990–1991

MSA	Black/white ratios of age-specific rates			Age-adjusted rates		
	15–24	25–34	35–44	Black	White	Ratio
MSAs WITH >1 MILLION TOTAL POPULATION IN 1980						
Anaheim	0.57	0.97	0.97	66.88	75.25	0.89
Atlanta	1.34	2.28	2.43	154.73	72.45	2.14
Baltimore	1.77	2.96	3.28	201.63	69.29	2.91
Boston	2.34	1.28	1.22	173.37	130.88	1.32
Buffalo	1.73	2.88	2.66	189.44	73.05	2.59
Chicago	2.07	3.26	3.00	211.33	73.07	2.89
Cincinnati	1.88	1.67	1.66	122.31	71.87	1.70
Cleveland	1.67	2.69	2.86	178.24	69.00	2.58
Columbus	1.43	2.42	1.98	137.46	67.95	2.02
Dallas	1.33	2.02	2.29	161.56	80.45	2.01
Denver	1.45	1.89	2.04	135.93	72.35	1.88
Detroit	1.73	2.88	1.97	196.67	91.54	2.15
Fort Lauderdale	1.40	3.09	2.60	231.07	90.95	2.54
Houston	1.31	2.07	2.09	176.80	93.41	1.89
Indianapolis	0.78	1.03	1.58	161.49	132.25	1.22
Kansas City	2.21	2.63	2.47	166.40	67.66	2.46
Los Angeles	1.29	1.67	1.74	173.47	106.78	1.62
Miami	2.05	3.45	3.18	253.92	82.40	3.08
Milwaukee	2.06	3.39	2.06	141.90	59.94	2.37
Minneapolis	1.00	1.33	1.51	128.56	95.16	1.35
Nassau-Suffolk	1.87	3.55	2.70	186.03	66.05	2.82
New Orleans	1.39	2.58	2.49	173.94	77.36	2.25
New York, NY	1.31	1.79	2.05	247.20	133.68	1.85
Newark	2.96	5.19	5.13	344.68	71.64	4.81
Philadelphia	1.70	2.40	2.38	170.88	75.05	2.28
Phoenix	1.76	2.74	1.59	155.17	79.82	1.94
Pittsburgh	1.32	2.50	2.70	172.80	70.45	2.45
Portland	0.36	2.58	2.33	130.20	65.69	1.98
Riverside	0.97	1.86	1.64	161.00	102.33	1.57
Sacramento	1.84	1.60	1.59	138.19	84.27	1.64
St. Louis	1.71	2.29	2.99	168.80	66.79	2.53
San Antonio	0.97	1.54	1.65	135.55	91.26	1.49
San Diego	1.22	1.80	2.02	151.16	83.69	1.81
San Jose	0.59	1.14	1.42	74.72	62.67	1.19
Seattle	0.68	3.40	1.74	114.92	60.11	1.91
Tampa	1.36	2.82	2.65	196.90	79.68	2.47
Washington, DC	1.99	3.48	2.95	162.66	55.99	2.91
MSAs WITH >150,000 BLACKS IN 1990						
Baton Rouge	1.40	2.79	1.88	168.19	81.71	2.06
Birmingham	0.78	2.01	2.32	179.72	97.02	1.85
Charlotte	0.99	2.84	2.91	182.97	73.43	2.49
Charlestown	1.26	2.19	2.10	174.08	88.04	1.98
Greensboro	1.17	2.57	2.62	175.83	76.86	2.29

(continued)

Table A-9. Black/white ratios of mortality rates for young adult females and age-adjusted mortality rates (ages 15–44 years) in 50 MSAs, 1990–1991 (Continued)

	Black/white ratios of age-specific rates			Age-adjusted rates		
MSA	15–24	25–34	35–44	Black	White	Ratio
Jackson, MS	0.61	1.78	1.91	134.60	90.74	1.48
Jacksonville	1.29	2.71	1.99	190.18	91.88	2.07
Memphis	2.13	2.82	2.61	194.27	75.35	2.58
Nashville	0.91	2.84	1.70	139.22	76.25	1.83
Norfolk	1.46	1.93	2.14	137.10	69.85	1.96
Oakland	1.61	2.29	2.52	180.82	80.40	2.25
Raleigh	2.09	2.43	2.92	145.49	55.60	2.62
Richmond	1.47	2.49	1.96	142.04	70.74	2.01

Table A-10. Mortality rates for men aged 45–54 and 55–64 years in 50 MSAs, 1990–1991

	Segregation	Whites		Blacks		Black/white ratio	
MSA	index	45–54	55–64	45–54	55–64	45–54	55–64
MSAs WITH > 1 MILLION TOTAL POPULATION IN 1980							
Anaheim	43	448.3	1,167.8	426.0	1,777.3	0.95	1.52
Atlanta	73	534.0	1,415.4	1,256.9	3,039.1	2.35	2.15
Baltimore	75	539.9	1,519.5	1,405.8	2,840.9	2.60	1.87
Boston	70	667.1	1,864.4	1,046.2	2,204.7	1.57	1.18
Buffalo	84	559.4	1,560.0	1,322.4	2,527.7	2.36	1.62
Chicago	87	594.1	1,509.9	1,569.2	2,852.8	2.64	1.89
Cincinnati	80	534.5	1,600.9	984.5	2,829.1	1.84	1.77
Cleveland	86	536.3	1,455.1	1,167.1	2,499.5	2.18	1.72
Columbus	71	517.7	1,522.6	1,009.9	2,331.7	1.95	1.53
Dallas	66	594.3	1,489.3	1,284.8	2,922.9	2.16	1.96
Denver	66	494.4	1,270.8	850.8	2,060.8	1.72	1.62
Detroit	89	523.7	1,465.7	1,363.1	2,566.0	2.60	1.75
Fort Lauderdale	73	678.9	1,435.1	1,010.0	2,555.9	1.49	1.78
Houston	69	655.2	1,644.0	1,259.9	2,654.5	1.92	1.61
Indianapolis	80	503.2	1,562.1	1,021.8	2,392.7	2.03	1.53
Kansas City	76	531.5	1,438.3	1,074.0	2,542.1	2.02	1.77
Los Angeles	71	744.1	1,532.8	1,273.7	2,525.8	1.71	1.65
Miami	75	670.3	1,465.2	1,327.7	2,505.4	1.98	1.71
Milwaukee	84	466.6	1,326.2	1,261.3	2,302.7	2.70	1.74
Minneapolis	65	398.0	1,176.7	1,218.7	2,520.8	3.06	2.14
Nassau-Suffolk	79	469.4	1,273.4	832.7	1,928.0	1.77	1.51
New Orleans	74	676.1	1,799.3	1,497.7	2,970.6	2.22	1.65
New York, NY	78	916.2	1,611.3	1,475.3	2,397.4	1.61	1.49
Newark	83	499.2	1,203.4	1,447.9	2,912.9	2.90	2.42
Philadelphia	82	540.8	1,481.3	1,391.7	2,732.7	2.57	1.84
Phoenix	51	565.0	1,423.2	913.2	2,188.4	1.62	1.54
Pittsburgh	75	624.6	1,513.3	1,241.8	2,438.2	1.99	1.61

(continued)

Table A-10. (Continued)

MSA	Segregation index	Whites 45–54	Whites 55–64	Blacks 45–54	Blacks 55–64	Black/white ratio 45–54	Black/white ratio 55–64
Portland	68	491.8	1,429.7	1,099.6	2,509.5	2.24	1.76
Riverside	49	732.5	1,679.9	896.1	1,912.6	1.22	1.14
Sacramento	58	602.2	1,482.2	1,030.9	1,986.3	1.71	1.34
St Louis	81	457.6	1,462.5	1,322.3	2,840.2	2.89	1.94
San Antonio	57	702.6	1,734.7	961.8	2,108.8	1.37	1.22
San Diego	59	567.9	1,335.9	828.7	2,112.7	1.46	1.58
San Jose	46	464.4	1,149.2	527.3	2,003.3	1.14	1.74
Seattle	60	430.5	1,168.4	858.0	2,252.3	1.99	1.93
Tampa	74	656.9	1,579.3	1,202.2	2,688.9	1.83	1.70
Washington, DC	68	400.9	1,154.8	1,149.9	2,402.9	2.87	2.08
MSAs WITH > 150,000 BLACKS IN 1990							
Baton Rouge	73	489.3	1,534.2	1,168.5	2,656.5	2.39	1.73
Birmingham	79	672.5	1,608.0	1,403.4	2,525.8	2.09	1.57
Charleston	58	639.8	1,537.3	1,270.8	2,918.2	1.99	1.90
Charlotte	65	587.6	1,565.1	1,456.0	2,940.7	2.48	1.88
Greensboro	68	557.1	1,386.3	1,422.2	2,546.3	2.55	1.84
Jackson, MS	75	562.4	1,533.3	1,297.3	2,525.3	2.31	1.65
Jacksonville	65	577.6	1,673.7	1,234.7	3,039.1	2.14	1.82
Memphis	76	506.2	1,515.2	1,350.3	2,913.5	2.67	1.92
Nashville	66	556.5	1,528.2	1,295.6	2,767.7	2.33	1.81
Norfolk	57	514.3	1,548.6	1,151.6	2,702.7	2.24	1.75
Oakland	69	524.1	1,370.9	1,325.9	2,585.8	2.53	1.89
Raleigh	57	410.2	1,313.8	1,413.4	2,594.8	3.45	1.97
Richmond	64	483.5	1,488.7	1,250.0	2,685.2	2.59	1.80

Table A-11. Prediction of mortality rate for blacks and black/white ratio of mortality rates for ages 45–54 and 55–64 years in 50 MSAs, 1990–1991

	Black mortality rate			B/W mortality ratio			
	Coefficient	t	p	Coefficient	t	p	
MEN							
AGES 45–54							
Poverty, black	0.723	1.67	0.101	B/W poverty	0.292	4.69	<0.001
Segregation	10.795	3.70	0.001	Segregation	0.005	0.74	0.465
Constant	227.780			Constant	0.728		
R^2	0.363			R^2	0.435		
AGES 55–64							
Poverty, black	1.213	1.90	0.064	B/W poverty	0.118	3.53	0.001
Segregation	8.940	2.08	0.043	Segregation	−0.002	−0.469	0.641
Constant	1,573.637			Constant	1.403		
R^2	0.218			R^2	0.223		
WOMEN							
AGES 45–54							
Poverty, black	0.225	1.16	0.251	B/W poverty	0.108	2.00	0.051
Segregation	3.912	3.00	0.004	Segregation	0.006	1.14	0.260
Constant	267.1			Constant	1.099		
R^2	0.250			R^2	0.168		
AGES 55–64							
Poverty, black	0.856	2.82	0.007	B/W poverty	0.041	1.38	0.174
Segregation	5.312	2.60	0.013	Segregation	0.008	2.55	0.014
Constant	830.06			Constant	1.023		
R^2	0.356			R^2	0.254		

Table A-12. Mortality rates for women ages 45–54 and 55–64 in 50 MSAs, 1990–1991

MSA	Segregation index 1990	White death rates 45–54	White death rates 55–64	Black death rates 45–54	Black death rates 55–64	B/W ratio 45–54	B/W ratio 55–64
MSAs WITH > 1 MILLION POPULATION IN 1980							
Anaheim	43	288.4	750.6	367.0	964.2	1.27	1.28
Atlanta	73	273.0	777.0	620.6	1,546.2	2.27	1.99
Baltimore	75	304.3	871.4	698.9	1,451.8	2.30	1.67
Boston	70	394.2	1,049.0	505.9	1,431.8	1.28	1.36
Buffalo	84	335.0	882.2	754.3	1,640.3	2.25	1.86
Chicago	87	319.9	877.2	741.1	1,557.5	2.32	1.78
Cincinati	80	356.4	940.7	609.2	1,535.7	1.71	1.63
Cleveland	86	311.6	851.6	591.9	1,406.5	1.90	1.65
Columbus	71	319.0	970.3	527.0	1,286.7	1.65	1.33
Dallas	66	284.5	825.5	643.5	1,594.8	2.26	1.93
Denver	66	266.0	750.0	419.0	1,317.8	1.58	1.76
Detroit	89	335.4	877.9	629.8	1,474.5	1.88	1.68
Fort Lauderdale	73	353.0	755.4	545.2	1,361.7	1.54	1.80
Houston	69	344.2	928.6	588.6	1,534.5	1.71	1.65
Indianapolis	80	327.3	848.1	492.7	1,528.1	1.51	1.80
Kansas City	76	302.4	791.0	588.9	1,483.3	1.95	1.88
Los Angeles	71	385.3	915.9	625.0	1,355.2	1.62	1.48
Miami	75	282.8	669.7	650.8	1,458.1	2.30	2.18
Milwaukee	84	277.7	756.6	480.1	1,372.7	1.73	1.81
Minneapolis	65	246.8	742.6	550.9	1,318.6	2.23	1.78
Nassau-Suffolk	79	281.3	760.7	534.0	1,228.9	1.90	1.62
New Orleans	74	362.2	888.7	639.7	1,685.9	1.77	1.90
New York, NY	78	409.7	915.9	615.8	1,295.5	1.50	1.41
Newark	83	276.2	736.5	723.0	1,508.4	2.62	2.05
Philadelphia	82	328.8	865.2	716.3	1,534.8	2.18	1.77
Phoenix	51	320.0	804.6	525.4	1,121.4	1.64	1.39
Pittsburgh	75	317.7	842.0	688.7	1,491.4	2.17	1.77
Portland	68	290.1	820.5	654.5	1,519.1	2.26	1.85
Riverside	49	424.7	999.9	568.3	1,689.6	1.34	1.69
Sacramento	58	365.1	951.1	496.9	1,450.0	1.36	1.52
St Louis	81	304.8	828.8	637.6	1,617.8	2.09	1.95
San Antonio	57	346.5	926.0	438.1	1,452.6	1.26	1.57
San Diego	59	351.3	809.7	582.4	1,276.9	1.66	1.58
San Jose	46	275.9	794.6	377.6	821.8	1.37	1.03
Seattle	60	266.0	791.4	440.5	1,311.6	1.66	1.66
Tampa	74	328.6	788.4	694.8	1,470.8	2.11	1.87
Washington, DC	68	217.2	724.1	613.2	1,384.6	2.82	1.91
MSAs WITH > 150,000 BLACKS IN 1990							
Baton Rouge	73	333.7	810.9	730.0	1,543.0	2.19	1.90
Birmingham	79	319.5	857.0	753.8	1,705.6	2.36	1.99
Charlotte	65	291.6	823.6	699.9	1,461.0	2.40	1.77
Charleston	58	300.3	832.4	639.4	1,342.0	2.13	1.61
Greensboro	68	287.0	817.0	582.3	1,372.2	2.03	1.68
Jackson, MS	75	281.1	762.1	539.0	1,468.7	1.92	1.93
Jacksonville	65	360.0	887.5	775.4	1,597.7	2.15	1.80

(continued)

Table A-12. Mortality rates for women ages 45–54 and 55–64 in 50 MSAs, 1990–1991 (Continued)

MSA	Segregation index 1990	White death rates 45–54	White death rates 55–64	Black death rates 45–54	Black death rates 55–64	B/W ratio 45–54	B/W ratio 55–64
Memphis	76	325.7	847.8	643.4	1,617.0	1.98	1.91
Nashville	66	315.4	817.4	650.4	1,473.2	2.06	1.80
Norfolk	57	284.6	866.8	626.6	1,441.2	2.20	1.66
Oakland	69	315.9	899.7	704.5	1,415.3	2.23	1.57
Raleigh	57	235.1	711.7	525.3	1,291.0	2.23	1.81
Richmond	64	297.7	893.3	605.0	1,377.3	2.03	1.54

Table A-13. Prediction of mortality rate for black and white males 15–44 years of age in 46 MSAs with data on total homicide rate by MSA

Variable	Blacks Coefficient	Blacks t	Blacks p	Whites Coefficient	Whites t	Whites p
Segregation index	6.373	5.28	<0.001	−0.936	−1.47	0.149
Poverty rate (race-specific)	−0.298	−1.68	0.101	1.189	4.14	<0.001
Total homicide rate	1.031	6.23	<0.001	0.395	3.76	0.001
Constant	−39.046			130.643		
Adjusted R²	0.643			0.489		

Table A-14. Characteristics of 33 MSAs used for analysis of black mortality rates (ages 15–44 years) in relation to black housing–neighborhood quality and total homicide rate

MSA	Segregation index	Black poverty	Occupied units with black householder				Total homicide rate
			Number of units (in 1,000s)	Lower quality housing	Lower quality neighborhood	1.01+ persons/ room	
MSAs WITH >1 MILLION TOTAL POPULATION IN 1980							
Anaheim	43	9.7	133	0.02	0.07	0.00	62
Atlanta	73	22.4	2,563	0.05	0.10	0.03	137
Baltimore	75	23.2	1,995	0.06	0.15	0.03	156
Boston	70	21.7	749	0.08	0.15	0.05	61
Buffalo	84	37.4	421	0.03	0.10	0.01	45
Chicago	87	30.0	4,591	0.07	0.21	0.06	156
Cincinnati	80	34.0	673	0.08	0.16	0.03	52
Cleveland	86	31.0	1,354	0.05	0.13	0.03	113
Columbus	71	28.9	536	0.06	0.15	0.02	80
Dallas	66	26.7	1,337	0.06	0.13	0.07	214
Denver	66	24.6	334	0.05	0.13	0.01	58
Detroit	89	33.0	3,195	0.07	0.17	0.02	163
Houston	69	27.9	2,255	0.06	0.13	0.05	211
Indianapolis	80	26.2	568	0.09	0.13	0.05	70
Kansas City	76	28.1	684	0.08	0.14	0.05	114
Los Angeles	71	21.2	3,478	0.06	0.15	0.05	199
Milwaukee	84	41.3	583	0.10	0.20	0.05	112
New Orleans	74	40.8	1,387	0.05	0.13	0.07	312
New York, NY	78	24.8	7,645	0.08	0.18	0.09	269
Philadelphia	82	25.5	2,940	0.04	0.17	0.04	132
Phoenix	51	27.4	215	0.07	0.11	0.07	82
Pittsburgh	75	35.9	618	0.07	0.19	0.03	33
Portland	68	29.3	121	0.08	0.17	0.02	44
St. Louis	81	31.3	1,383	0.06	0.15	0.06	129
San Antonio	57	26.4	288	0.07	0.11	0.03	179
San Diego	59	21.3	492	0.06	0.13	0.07	86
San Jose	46	12.7	174	0.05	0.09	0.01	38
Seattle	60	21.7	427	0.04	0.06	0.03	48
Washington, DC	68	12.6	3,575	0.05	0.11	0.02	174
MSAs WITH > 150,000 BLACKS IN 1990							
Birmingham	79	31.4	892	0.05	0.10	0.06	194
Memphis	76	34.9	1,310	0.07	0.11	0.08	229
Norfolk	57	25.1	1,290	0.06	0.08	0.03	120
Oakland	69	21.1	1,451	0.05	0.14	0.03	124

Table A-15. Correlation coefficients between black housing and neighborhood quality variables for 33 MSAs (blacks only)

	Persons/ room 1.01+	Lower quality housing	Segregation Lower quality neighborhood	Black index, 1990	Black poverty 1990
Persons/room	—	0.4425*	0.2623	0.2166	0.3232
Housing	0.4425*	—	0.6592†	0.3931	0.4683*
Neighborhood	0.2623	0.6592†	—	0.6286†	0.4595*
Segregation	0.2166	0.3931	0.6286†	—	0.6620†
Black poverty	0.3232	0.4683*	0.4595*	0.6620†	—

One-tailed Significance test: *0.01, †0.001.

Table A-16. Multiple regression analysis of mortality rate for black men 15–44 (age-standardized rate) in 33 MSAs, 1990–1991*

Variable	Coefficient	t	p
Segregation index, 1990	3.993	2.69	0.012
Homicides (1990)	1.110	5.97	<0.001
Neighborhood quality	6.922	1.51	0.143
Constant	−64.492		
Adjusted R²	0.693		

*Neighborhood quality: Number of occupied units with black householder where respondent rated the neighborhood as low (1–4 on a 10-point scale) divided by the total number of such occupied units. This figure ranged from 0.0609 to 0.2091. Homicides: Homicide rate (FBI, 1990). Variables not included: property crime rate; black poverty rate.

Table A-17. Multiple regression analysis of total age-adjusted death rates for 1990 in 50 MSAs: statistical significance (p values) of independent variables

	p Value		
	Cardiovascular	Nephritis	Homicide
Percent black	<0.001*	0.002*	<0.001*
Black/white poverty	0.553	0.607	0.003*
Segregation index	0.010*	0.055	0.093
Adjusted R²	0.387	0.354	0.498

*Statistically significant. The black/white poverty rate ratio was negatively associated with homicide rates when the other variables were included in the model.

References

Aaby P, Bukh J, Lisse IM et al. Overcrowing and intensive exposure as determinants of measles mortality. *Am J Epidemiol* 1984;120:49–63.

Ader R, Cohen N, Felten D. Psychoneuroimmunology: Interactions between the nervous system and the immune system. *Lancet* 1995;345:99–103.

Adler NE, Boyce WT, Chesney MA et al. Socioeconomic inequalities in health: No easy solution. *JAMA* 1993;269:3140–3145.

Adler NE, Boyce WT, Chesney MA et al. Socioeconomic status and health: The challenge of the gradient. *Am Psychol* 1994;49:15–24.

Afifi AA, Clark V. *Computer-Aided Multivariate Analysis*. Belmont, CA: Lifetime Learning Publications, 1984.

Allport GW. *The Nature of Prejudice*. 25th Anniversary Edition. Reading, MA: Addison-Wesley, 1969.

American Medical Association. Black–white disparities in health care. *JAMA* 1990; 263:2344–2346.

American Public Health Association. *Healthy Communities 2000: Model Standards*. 3rd Ed. Washington, DC: American Public Health Association, 1991.

Andrulis DP, Acuff KL, Weiss KB et al. Public hospitals and health care reform: Choices and challenges. *Am J Public Health* 1996;86:162–165.

Anon. The underclass. *Lancet* 1990;1:1312–1313.

Anon. Not a classless society. *Lancet* 1991;338:1116.

Anon. Against the culture of contentment. *Lancet* 1993;342:1373–1374.

Anon. Less equal than others. *Lancet* 1994;343:805–806.

Anon. New way to measure poverty advocated in National Research Council report. *Nation's Health* 1995a, July, p 11.

Anon. The unequal, the achievable, and the champion. *Lancet* 1995b;345:1061–1062.

Antonovsky A, Bernstein J. Social class and infant mortality. *Soc Sci Med* 1977;11:453–470.

Armstead CA, Lawler KA, Gorden G, Cross J, Gibbons J. Relationship of racial stressors to blood pressure responses and anger expression in black college students. *Health Psychol* 1989;8:541–556.

Attinasi JJ. Racism, language variety, and urban U.S. minorities: Issues in bilingualism and bidialectalism. In Gregory S; Sanjek R (eds); *Race*. New Brunswick, NJ: Rutgers University Press, 1994, pp 319–347.

Ayanian JZ. Race, class, and the quality of medical care. *JAMA* 1994;271:1207–1208.

163

Baldwin J. *The Fire Next Time*. New York: Dial Press, 1963.

Bane MJ, Elwood DT. One fifth of the nation's children: Why are they poor? *Science* 1989;245:1047–1053.

Baquet CR, Horm JW, Gibbs T et al. Socioeconomic factors and cancer incidence among blacks and whites. *JNCI* 1991;83:551–557.

Barefoot JC, Larsen S, von der Lieth L et al. Hostility, incidence of acute myocardial infarction, and mortality in a sample of older Danish men and women. *Am J Epidemiol* 1995;142:477–484.

Barker DJP, Coggon D, Osmond C et al. Poor housing in childhood and high rates of stomach cancer in England and Wales. *Br J Cancer* 1990;61:575–578.

Basu A, Namboodiri KK, Weitkamp LR et al. Morphology, serology, dermatoglyphics, and microevolution of some village populations in Haiti, West Indies. *Hum Biol* 1976;48:245–269.

Bayer R, Wilkinson D. Directly observed therapy for tuberculosis: History of an idea. *Lancet* 1995;345:1545–1547.

Becker TM, Wiggins CL, Key CR, Samet JM. Symptoms, signs, and ill-defined conditions: A leading cause of death among minorities. *Am J Epidemiol* 1990;131:664–668.

Berry JW, Kim U, Minde T et al. Comparative studies of acculturation stress. *Int Migration Rev* 1987;21:491–511.

Besharov DJ. Poverty, welfare dependency, and the underclass. In Darby MR (ed): *Reducing poverty in America: Views and Approaches*. Thousand Oaks, CA: Sage Publications, 1996, pp 13–56.

Bindman AB, Grumbach K, Osmond D et al. Preventable hospitalizations and access to health care. *JAMA* 1995;274:305–311.

Bird ST, Baumann KE. The relationship between structural and health services variables and state-level infant mortality in the United States. *Am J Public Health* 1995;85:26–29.

Birkhead GS, LeBaron CW, Parsons P et al. The immunization of children enrolled in the Special Supplemental Food Program for Women, Infants, and Children (WIC). *JAMA* 1995;274:312–316.

Black Research Working Group. *Inequalities in Health*. The Black report. London: Department of Health and Social Security, 1980.

Blendon RJ, Scheck AC, Donelan K et al. How white and African Americans view their health and social problems: Different experiences, different expectations. *JAMA* 1995;273:341–346.

Blumenthal DS, Sung J, Caotes R et al. Recruitment and retention of subjects for a longitudinal cancer prevention study in an inner-city black community. *Health Services Res* 1995;30(Part II):197–205.

Blustein J. The reliability of racial classifications in hospital discharge abstract data. *Am J Public Health* 1994;84:1018–1021.

Boas F. *Race and Democratic Society*. 1945. Reprinted, New York: Biblo and Tannen, 1969.

Botha JL, Bradshaw D, Gonin R et al. The distribution of health needs and services in South Africa. *Soc Sci Med* 1988;26:845–851.

Bouchardy C, Mirra AP, Khlat M et al. Ethnicity and cancer risk in São Paulo, Brazil. *Cancer Epidemiol Biomarkers Prev* 1991;1:21–27.

Braveman P, Egerter S, Edmonston F et al. Racial/ethnic differences in the likelihood of cesarean delivery, California. *Am J Public Health* 1995;85:625–630.

Brownson RC, Smith CA, Pratt M et al. Preventing cardiovascular disease through community-based risk reduction: The Bootheel Heart Health Project. *Am J Public Health* 1996;86:206–213.

Bryant B, Mohai P (eds). *Race and the Incidence of Environmental Hazards: A Time for Discourse.* Boulder, CO: Westview Press, 1992.

Bryce-Laporte RS. Voluntary immigration and continuing encounters between blacks: The post-quincentenary challenge. *Ann Am Acad Polit Soc Sci* 1993;530:28–41.

Bullard RD. Solid waste sites and the black Houston community. *Sociol Inquiry* 1983;53:273–288.

Butkus DE, Meydrich EF, Raju SS. Racial differences in the survival of cadaveric renal allografts. *N Engl J Med* 1992;327:840–845.

Cabral H, Fried LE, Levenson S et al. Foreign-born and US-born black women: Differences in health behaviors and birth outcomes. *Am J Public Health* 1990; 80:70–72.

Carleton RA, Lasater TM, Assaf AR et al. The Pawtucket Heart Health program: Community changes in cardiovascular risk factors and projected disease risk. *Am J Public Health* 1995;85:777–785.

Carr W, Szapiro N, Heisler T et al. Sentinel health events as indicators of unmet needs. *Soc Sci Med* 1989;29:705–714.

Centers for Disease Control and Prevention. Increasing breast cancer screening among the medically underserved—Dade County, Florida, September 1987–March 1991. *MMWR* 1991;40:261–263.

Centers for Disease Control and Prevention. Differences in infant mortality between blacks and whites—United States, 1980–1991. *MMWR* 1994;43:288–289.

Centers for Disease Control and Prevention. Block grant may imperil future of DOT strategy. *Health Lett CDC* 1995, April 10, p 5.

Chakraborty R. Gene admixture in human populations: Models and predictions. *Yearbk Phys Anthropol* 1986;29:1–43.

Chakraborty R, Kamboh MI, Nwankwo M et al. Caucasian genes in American blacks: New data. *Am J Hum Genet* 1992;50:145–155.

Charatz-Litt C. A chronicle of racism: The effects of the white medical community on black health. *J Natl Med Assoc* 1992;84:717–725.

Charlton BG. Is inequality bad for the national health? *Lancet* 1994;343:221–222.

Childe VG. *Man Makes Himself.* New York: Mentor Nooks, 1951.

Collins JW Jr, David RJ. Differences in neonatal mortality by race, income, and prenatal care. *Ethnicity Dis* 1992;2:18–26.

Collins JW, David RJ. Race and birthweight in biracial infants. *Am J Public Health* 1993;83:1125–1129.

Comstock GW. An epidemiologic study of blood pressure levels in a biracial community in the southern Unites States. *Am J Hyg* 1957;65:271–315. Reprinted in *Am J Epidemiol*, 1995;141:584–628.

Connor MK. *What is Cool? Understanding Black Manhood in America.* New York: Crown, 1995.

Cooper RS. Health and the social status of blacks in the United States. *Ann Epidemiol* 1993;3:137–144.

Cooper RS. A case study in the use of race and ethnicity in public health surveillance. *Public Health Rep* 1994;109:46–52.

Cowie MR, Fahrenbruch CE, Cobb LA et al. Out-of-hospital cardiac arrest: Racial differences in outcome in Seattle. *Am J Public Health* 1993;83:955–959.

Crawford SL, McGraw SA, Smith KW et al. Do blacks and whites differ in their use of health care for symptoms of coronary heart disease? *Am J Public Health* 1994; 84:957–964.

Crews DE, Bindon JR. Ethnicity as a taxonomic category in biomedical and biosocial research. *Ethnic Dis* 1991;1:42–49.

Cuellar J, Harris LC, Jasso R. An acculturation scale for Mexican American normal and clinical populations. *Hispan J Behav Sci* 1980;2:199–217.

Darby MR. *Reducing Poverty in America: Views and Approaches.* Thousand Oaks, CA: Sage, 1996.

Davidson LL, Durkin MS, Kuhn L et al. The impact of the Safe Kids/Health Neighborhoods Injury Prevention Program in Harlem, 1988 through 1991, *Am J Public Health* 1994;84:580–586.

Davis FJ. *Who is Black?* University Park, PA: Pennsylvania State University Press, 1991, p 25.

Day JC. *Population Projections of the United States, by Age, Sex, Race, and Hispanic Origin: 1993 to 2050.* U.S. Bureau of the Census, Current Population Reports, P25-1104. Washington, DC: U.S. Government Printing Office, 1993.

Dean M, Stephens C, Winkler C et al. Polymorphic admixture typing in human ethnic populations. *Am J Hum Genet* 1994;55:788–808.

DeVita VT Jr. Cancer prevention awareness program: Targeting black Americans. *Public Health Rep* 1985;100:253–254.

Diez-Roux AV, Nieto J, Tyroler HA et al. Social inequalities and atherosclerosis: The Atherosclerosis Risk in Communities Study. *Am J Epidemiol* 1995;141:960–972.

Dooley AR Jr. Review of *From Consumption to Tuberculosis—A Documentary History,* by Rosenkrantz BG (ed). *Health Values* 1995;19:57–59.

Dougherty CJ. *American Health Care. Realities, Rights, and Reforms.* New York: Oxford University Press, 1988.

Dressler WW. Health in the African American community: Accounting for health inequalities. *Med Anthropol Q* 1993;7:325–345.

Dressler WW. Social identity and arterial blood pressure in the African-American community. *Ethnicity Dis* 1996;6:176–189.

Dubay LC, Norton SA, Moon M. Medicaid expansions for pregnant women and infants: Easing hospitals' uncompensated care burdens? *Inquiry* 1995;32:332–344.

Du Bois WEB. *The Philadelphia Negro: A Social Study.* Originally published in 1899 by University of Pennsylvania Press. Reprinted by Millwood, NY: Kraus-Thomson, 1973.

Duncan GJ, Hill MS, Hoffman SD. Welfare dependence within and across generations. *Science* 1988;239:467–471.

Duneier M. *Slim's Table: Race, Respectability, and Masculinity.* Chicago: University of Chicago Press, 1992.

DuRant RH, Cadenhead C, Pendergast RA et al. Factors associated with the use of violence among urban black adolescents. *Am J Public Health* 1994;84:612–617.

Durkin MS, Davisdon LL, Kuhn L et al. Low income neighborhoods and the risk of pediatric injury: A small-area analysis in northern Manhattan. *Am J Public Health* 1994;84:587–592.

Earls F, Powell J. Patterns of substance abuse in inner-city adolescent medical patients. *Yale J Biol Med* 1988;61:233–242.

Eddy DM. What care is "essential"? What services are "basic"? *JAMA* 1991;265:782–788.

Edwards CH, Cole OJ, Oyemade UJ et al. Maternal stress and pregnancy outcomes in a prenatal clinic population. *J Nutr* 1994a;124:1006S–1021S.

Edwards CH, Knight EM, Johnson AA et al. African American women and their pregnancies: Demographic profile, methodology, and biochemical correlates during the course of pregnancy. *J Nutr* 1994b;124:917S–926S.

Escarce JJ, Epstein KR, Colby DC, Schwartz JS. Racial differences in the elderly's use of medical procedures and diagnostic tests. *Am J Public Health* 1993;83:948–954.

Ewbank DC. History of black mortality and health before 1940. *Milbank Mem Fund Q* 1987;65(Suppl. 1):100–128.

Ezekiel RS. *The Racist Mind*. New York: Viking, 1995.

Fanon F. The fact of blackness. Originally published in French, 1952 by Paladin. Reprinted in Donald J, Rattansi A (eds): *"Race," Culture and Difference*. London: Sage Publications, 1992, pp 220–240.

Farley R. Residential segregation of social and economic groups among blacks, 1970–1980. In Jencks C, Peterson PE. *The Urban Underclass*. Washington, DC: The Brookings Institution, 1991, pp 274–298.

Farley R, Frey WH. Changes in the segregation of whites from blacks during the 1980s: Small steps toward a more integrated society. *Am Sociol Rev* 1994;59:23–45.

Farley R, Frey WH. Changes in the Segregation of Whites From Blacks During the 1980's: Small Steps Toward a More Racially Integrated Society. Ann Arbor, MI: Population Studies Center, University of Michigan, Research Report 92-257, 1992.

Feagin JR. The continuing significance of race: Antiblack discrimination in public places. *Am Sociol Rev* 1991;56:101–116.

Federal Bureau of Investigation. *Uniform Crime Reports, 1990*. Washington, DC: U.S. Government Printing Office, 1991.

Feingold E. The defeat of health care reform: Misplaced mistrust in government. *Am J Public Health* 1995;85:1619–1622.

Feldman JJ, Makuc DM, Kleinman JC, Cornoni-Huntley J. National trends in educational differentials in mortality. *Am J Epidemiol* 1989;129:919–933.

Felix-Ortiz M, Newcomb MD, Myers H. A multidimensional measure of cultural identity for Latino and Latina adolescents. *Hispan J Behav Sci* 1994;16:99–115.

Firebaugh G, Davis KE. Trends in antiblack prejudice, 1972–1984: Region and cohort effects. *Am J Sociol* 1988;94:251–272.

Firshein J. Number of black applicants to U.S. medical schools falls. *Lancet* 1995; 346:1286.

Fix M, Struyk RJ (eds). *Clear and Convincing Evidence: Measurement of Discrimination in America*. Latham, MD: Urban Institute Press, 1993.

Fong RL. Violence as a barrier to compliance for the hypertensive urban African American. *J Natl Med Assoc* 1995;87:203–207.

Ford ES, Cooper RS. Racial/ethnic differences in health care utilization of cardiovascular procedures: A review of the evidence. *Health Serv Res* 1995;30:237–251.

Foster HW, Jr, Thomas DJ, Semenya KA et al. Low birthweight in African-Americans: Does intergenerational well-being improve outcome? *J Natl Med Assoc* 1993; 516–520.

Frankel D. Tuberculosis decreases in New York. *Lancet* 1994;343:788.

Frankel D. New York's TB decline continues. *Lancet* 1995;345:783.

Franks P, Clancy CM, Gold MR et al. Health insurance and subjective health status: Data from the 1987 National Medical Expenditure Survey. *Am J Public Health* 1993;83:1295–1299.

Freedman DA. Adjusting the 1990 census. *Science* 1991;252:1233–1236.

Freehling WW. *The Reintegration of American History: Slavery and the Civil War.* New York: Oxford University Press, 1994.

Freeman HP. Poverty, race, racism, and survival *Ann Epidemiol* 1993;3:145–149.

Freidenberg J. Lower income urban enclaves. Introduction. *Ann NY Acad Sci* 1995; 749:1–40.

Freund DA, Hurley RE. Medicaid managed care: Contribution to issues of health reform. *Annu Rev Public Health* 1995;16:473–495.

Frieden TR. Tuberculosis control and social change. *Am J Public Health* 1994;84:1721–1723.

Fruchter RG, Nayeri K, Remy JC et al. Cervix and breast cancer incidence in immigrant Caribbean women. *Am J Public Health* 1990;80:722–724.

Fuchs LH. *The American Kaleidoscope: Race, Ethnicity, and the Civic Culture.* Hanover: University Press of America, 1990.

Fuchs LH. An agenda for tomorrow: Immigration policy and ethnic policies. *Ann Am Acad Polit Soc Sci* 1993;530:171–186.

Galbraith JK. *The Culture of Contentment.* Boston: Houghton Mifflin, 1992.

Galishoff S. *Newark: The Nation's Unhealthiest City, 1832–1895.* New Brunswick, NJ: Rutgers University Press, 1988.

Gamble VN. *Making a Place for Ourselves: The Black Hospital Movement, 1920–1945.* New York: Oxford University Press, 1995.

Gans HJ (ed). *Sociology in America.* Newbury Park, CA: Sage Publications, 1990.

Gans HJ. *People, Plans and Policies. Essays on Poverty, Racism, and Other National Urban Problems.* New York: Columbia University Press, 1993.

Gates-Williams J, Jackson MN, Jenkins-Monroe V, Williams LR. The business of preventing African-American infant mortality. *West J Med* 1992;157:350–356.

Glassman PA, Bell RM, Tranquada RE. The 1966 enactment of Medicare: Its effect on discharges from Los Angeles County–operated hospitals. *Am J Public Health* 1994;84:1325–1327.

Glazer N. Is assimilation dead? *Ann Am Acad Polit Soc Sci* 1993;530:122–136.

Gleiberman L, Harburg E, Frone MR et al. Skin colour, measures of socioeconomic status and blood pressure among blacks in Erie County, NY. *Ann Hum Biol* 1995;22:69–73.

Goldberg AI, Kirschenbaum A. Black newcomers to Israel: Contact situations and social distance. *Sociol Soc Res* 1989;74:52–57.

Greenland S, Robins J. Ecologic studies—biases, misconceptions, and counterexamples. *Am J Epidemiol* 1994a;139:747–760.

Greenland S, Robins J. Accepting the limits of ecologic studies: Drs. Greenland and Robins reply to Drs. Piantadosi and Cohen. *Am J Epidemiol* 1994b;139:769–771.

Greenstein R. Universal and targeted approaches to relieving poverty: An alternative view. In Jencks C, Peterson PE (eds): *The Urban Underclass.* Washington, DC: Brookings Institution, 1991, pp 437–459.

Griffin JH. *Black Like Me.* Updated. New York: Penguin, 1976.

Grulich AE, Swerdlow AJ, Head J et al. Cancer mortality in African and Caribbean migrants to England and Wales. *Br J Cancer* 1992;66:905–911.

Guralnick JM, Land KC, Blazer D et al. Educational status and life expectancy among older blacks and whites. *N Engl J Med* 1993;329:110–116.

Haan M, Kaplan GA, Camacho T. Poverty and health: Prospective study from the Alameda County study. *Am J Epidemiol* 1987;125:989–998.

Hackbarth DP, Silvestri B, Cosper W. Tobacco and alcohol billboards in 50 Chicago neighborhoods: Marker segmentation to sell dangerous products to the poor. *J Public Health Policy* 1995;16:213–230.

Hacker A. *Two Nations: Black and White, Separate, Hostile, Unequal.* New York: Charles Scribner's Sons, 1992.

Hacker A. *Two Nations: Black and White, Separate, Hostile, Unequal.* New York: Ballantine Books, 1995.

Hagoel L, Van-Raalte R, Kalekin-Fishman D et al. Psychosocial and medical factors in pregnancy outcomes: A case study of Israeli women. *Soc Sci Med* 1995;40:567–571.

Hahn RA, Mulinare J, Teutsch SM. Inconsistencies in coding of race and ethnicity between birth and death in US infants. *JAMA* 1992;267:259–263.

Hahn RA, Stroup DF. Race and ethnicity in public health surveillance: Criteria for the scientific use of social categories. *Public Health Rep* 1994;109:7–15.

Hahn RA, Teutsch SM, Rothenberg RB, Marks JS. Excess deaths from nine chronic diseases in the United States, 1986. *JAMA* 1990;264:1654–2659.

Hall C. "Models that Work" give lessons in providing primary care. *The Nation's Health* February 1996, p 8.

Hallinan MT, Williams RA. Interracial friendship choices in secondary schools. *Am Sociol Rev* 1989;54:67–78.

Hamilton DP. Census adjustment battle heats up. *Science* 1990;248:807–808.

Hannan EL, Kilburn H, O'Donnell JF et al. Interracial access to selected cardiac procedures for patients hospitalized with coronary artery disease in New York State. *Med Care* 1991;430–441.

Harrison FV. Racial and gender inequalities in health and health care. *Med Anthropol Q* 1994;8:90–95.

Harrison FV. The persistent power of "race" in the cultural and political economy of racism. *Annu Rev Anthropol* 1995;24:47–74.

Hayes-Bautista DE, Schink WO, Hayes-Bautista M. Latinos in the 1992 Los Angeles riots: A behavioral sciences perspective. *Hispan J Behav Sci* 1993;15:427–448.

Hazuda HP, Stern MP, Haffner SM. Acculturation and assimilation among Mexican-Americans: Scales and population-based data. *Soc Sci Q* 1988;69:687–706.

Helmer DC, Ragland DR, Syme SL. Hostility and coronary artery disease. *Am J Epidemiol* 1991;133:112–122.

Helms JE (ed). *Black and White Racial Identity: Theory, Research and Practice.* New York: Greenwood Press, 1990.

Henderson LA, Lerner M. Economic status, race, and mortality in Baltimore City, 1982–89. In National Center for Health Statistics Proceedings of the 1991 Public Health Conference on Records and Statistics, PHS 92-1214, 1992, pp 527–531.

Henry CP. *Culture and African American Politics.* Bloomington: University of Indiana Press, 1990.

Hogue CJR, Hargreaves MA. Class, race, and infant mortality in the United States. *Am J Public Health* 1993;83:9–12.

Holden C. African-American longevity. *Science* 1994;266:1482.

Holtzman NA. Science and the quiet art. Review of *The Role of Medical Research in Health Care,* by D. Weatherall. *Lancet* 1995;345:1097–1098.

hooks b. *Killing Rage: Ending Racism.* New York: Henry Holt, 1995.

Hunt WM. Measuring race and ethnicity is complex and controversial. Statement made in testimony before the Subcommittee on Census, Statistics and Postal Personnel, U.S. House of Representatives. April 13, 1993. Washington, DC: U.S. General Accounting Office.

Imbroscio D, Orr M, Ross T et al. Baltimore and the human investment challenge. In Wagner FW, Joder TE, Mumphrey AJ Jr (eds); *Urban Revitalization: Policies and Programs.* Thousand Oaks, CA: Sage, 1995, pp 38–68.

Jackson FLC. The bioanthropological context of disease. *Am J Kidney Dis* 1993;21 (Suppl 1):10–14.

Jackson JS, McCullough WR, Gurin G et al. Race identity. In Jackson JS (ed): *Life in Black America.* Newbury Park, CA: Sage, 1992, pp 238–253.

Jackson WA. *Gunnar Myrdal and America's Conscience. Social Engineering and Racial Liberalism, 1938–1987.* Chapel Hill, NC: University of North Carolina Press, 1990, p 296.

James SA, Keenan NL, Strogatz DS et al. Socioeconomic status, John Henryism, and blood pressure in black adults: The Pitt County Study. *Am J Epidemiol* 1992; 135:59–67.

James SA, Strogatz DS, Wing SB, Ramsey DL. Socioeconomic status, John Henryism, and hypertension in blacks and whites. *Am J Epidemiol* 1987;126:664–673.

Jargowsky PA, Bane MJ. Ghetto poverty on the United States, 1970–1980. In Jencks C, Peterson PE (eds): *The Urban Underclass.* Washington, DC: The Brookings Institution, 1991, pp 235–273.

Jaynes GD, Williams RM Jr (eds): *A Common Destiny: Blacks and American Society.* Washington, DC: National Academy Press, 1989.

Jencks C. Is the American underclass growing? In Jencks C, Peterson PE (eds): *The Urban Underclass.* Washington, DC: The Brookings Institution, 1991, pp 28–100.

Jencks C. *Rethinking Social Policy: Race, Poverty and the Underclass.* New York: Harper-Collins, 1993, p 200.

Jencks C, Peterson PE (eds): *The Urban Underclass.* Washington, DC: Brookings Institution, 1991.

Johnson BL, Coulberson SL. Environmental epidemiologic issues and minority health. *Ann Epidemiol* 1993;3:175–180.

Johnson JH Jr. The real issues for reducing poverty. In Darby MR (ed): *Reducing Poverty in America.* Thousand Oaks, CA: Sage, 1996, pp 337–363.

Joint Center for Political Studies. *A Policy Framework for Racial Justice.* Washington, DC: Joint Center for Political Studies, 1983.

Jones CP, LaVeist TA, Lillie-Blanton M. "Race" in the epidemiologic literature: An examination of the *American Journal of Epidemiology, 1921–1990. Am J Epidemiol* 1991;134:1079–1084.

Jones DR, Harrell JP, Morris-Prather CE et al. Affective and physiological responses to racism: The roles of Afrocentrism and mode of presentation. *Ethnicity Dis* 1996;6:109–122.

Jones JM. The concept of racism and its changing reality. In Bowser BJ, RG Hunt (eds): *Impacts of Racism on White Americans.* Beverly Hills, CA: Sage, 1981, pp 27–49.

Joyce T, Racine AD. An update on New York City's dramatic increase in low birthweights. *Am J Public Health* 1993;83:109–111.

Kahn KL, Pearson ML, Harrison ER, Desmond KA, Rogers WH, Rubenstein LV, Brook RH, Keeler EB. Health care for black and poor hospitalized Medicare patients. *JAMA* 1994:271:1169–1174.

Kalkstein LS. Lessons from a very hot summer. *Lancet* 1995;346:857–859.

Kaufmann PG, Parker SR, Lenfant C. Behavioral and biomedical research: A partnership for better health. *Psychosom Med* 1994;56:87–89.

Keith VM, Herring C. Skin tone and stratification in the black community. *Am J Sociol* 1991;97:760–778.

Kelso WA. *Poverty and the Underclass.* New York: New York University Press, 1994.

Kerner O (Chairman). *Report of the National Advisory Commission on Civil Disorders.* Washington, DC: U.S. Government Printing Office, 1968.

Khoury MJ, Beaty TH. Applications of the case–control method in genetic epidemiology. *Epidemiol Rev* 1994;16:134–150.

King G. Institutional racism and the medical/health complex: A conceptual analysis. *Ethnicity Dis* 1996,6:30–46.

King G, Bendel R. A statistical model estimating the number of African-American physicians in the United States. *J Natl Med Assoc* 1994;86:264–272.

Kinchen K, Wright JD. Hypertension management in health care for the homeless clinics: Results from a survey. *Am J Public Health* 1991;81:1163–1165.

Kitagawa EM, Hauser PM. *Differential Mortality in the United States: A Study in Socioeconomic Epidemiology.* Cambridge, MA: Harvard University Press, 1973.

Klag MJ, Whelton PK, Coresh J et al. The association of skin color with blood pressure in U.S. blacks with low socioeconomic status. *JAMA* 1991;265:599–602.

Klevens RM, Margules A, Cashman SB, Fulmer HS. Transforming a neighborhood health center into a community-oriented primary care practice. *Am J Prev Med* 1992;8:62–65.

Kliegman RM. Neonatal technology, perinatal survival, social consequences, and the perinatal paradox. *Am J Public Health* 1995;909–913.

Kogan MD, Kotelchuck M, Alexander GR et al. Racial disparities in reported prenatal care advice from health care providers. *Am J Public Health* 1994;84:82–88.

Krieger N. Shades of difference: Theoretical underpinnings of the medical controversy on black/white differences in the United States, 1830–1870. *Int J Health Services* 1987;17:259–278.

Krieger N. Racial and gender discrimination: Risk factors for high blood pressure? *Soc Sci Med* 1989;30:1273–1281.

Krieger N. Overcoming the absence of socioeconomic data in medical records: Validation and application of census-based methodology. *Am J Public Health* 1992; 92:703–710.

Krieger N, Fee E. Social class: The missing link in U.S. health data. *Int J Health Services* 1994;24:25–44.

Krieger N, Rowley DL. Re: "Race, family income, and low birth weight." *Am J Epidemiol* 1992;136:501.

Kuller LH. Epidemiology and health policy. *Am J Epidemiol* 1988;127:2–16.

Kuller LH. Invited commentary on "An Epidemiologic Study of Blood Pressure Levels in a Biracial Community in the Southern United States." *Am J Epidemiol* 1995;141:583.

Kumanyika S. Obesity in black women. *Epidemiol Rev* 1987;9:31–50.

Kunst AE, Mackenbach JP. The size of mortality differences associated with educational level in nine industrialized countries. *Am J Public Health* 1994;84:932–937.

Landry B. *The New Black Middle Class.* Berkeley: University of California Press, 1987.

Lane DS, Polednak AP, Burg MA. Breast cancer screening practices among users of county-funded health centers vs women in the entire community. *Am J Public Health* 1992;82:199–203.

Lang DM, Polansky M. Pattern of asthma mortality in Philadelphia from 1969 to 1991. *N Engl J Med* 1994;331:1542–1546.

LaVeist TA. Linking residential segregation to the infant-mortality race disparity in U.S. cities. *Sociol Soc Res* 1989;73:90–94.

LaVeist TA. The political empowerment and health status of African-Americans: Mapping a new territory. *Am J Sociol* 1992;97:1080–1095.

LaVeist TA. Segregation, poverty, and empowerment: Health consequences for African Americans. *Milbank Q* 1993;71:41–64.

Lemann N. *The Promised Land.* New York: Vintage, 1992.

Leuchtenburg WE. *Franklin D. Roosevelt and the New Deal.* New York: Harper and Row, 1963.

Lewis CE, Racyynski JM, Heath GW et al. Physical activity of public housing residents in Birmingham, Alabama. *Am J Public Health* 1993;83:1016–1020.

Lewis DL. *W.E.B. DuBois: Biography of a Race, 1868–1919.* New York: Henry Holt, 1993.

Lewis O. The culture of poverty. *Sci Am* 1966;215:19–25.

Liberatos P, Link GB, Kelsey LJ. The measurement of social class in epidemiology. *Epidemiol Rev* 1988;10:87–121.

Lichter DT. Racial differences in underemployment in American cities. *Am J Sociol* 1988;93:771–792.

Lieberman E, Ryan KJ, Monson RR, Shoenbaum SC. Risk factors accounting for racial differences in the rate of premature birth. *N Engl J Med* 1987;317:743–748.

Lieberson S. *A Piece of the Pie.* Berkeley, CA: University of California Press, 1990.

Lillie-Blanton M, Anthony JC, Schuster CR. Probing the meaning of racial/ethnic group comparisons in crack cocaine smoking. *JAMA* 1995;269:993–997.

Link BG, Susser E, Stueve A et al. Lifetime and five-year prevalence of homelessness in the United States. *Am J Public Health* 1994;84:1907–1912.

Littlefield A, Lieberman L, Reynolds LT. Redefining race: The potential demise of a concept in physical anthropology. *Curr Anthropol* 1982;23:641–655.

Loury G. The impossible dilemma. *The New Republic.* January 1, 1966, pp 21–25.

MacMahon B, Pugh TF. *Epidemiology: Principles and Methods.* Boston: Little-Brown, 1970.

Manfredi C, Lacey L, Warnecke R et al. Smoking-related behavior, beliefs, and social environment of young black women in subsidized public housing in Chicago. *Am J Public Health* 1992;82:267–272.

Marmot MG, Kogevinas M, Elston MA. Social/economic status and disease. *Annu Rev Public Health* 1987;8:111–135.

Massey DS. Latinos, poverty, and the underclass: A new agenda for research. *Hispan J Behav Sci* 1993;15:449–475.

Massey DS, Denton NA. Trends in residential segregation of blacks, Hispanics, and Asians: 1970–1980. *Am Sociol Rev* 1987;52:802–825.

Massey DS, Denton NA. *American Apartheid: Segregation and the Making of the Underclass.* Cambridge, MA: Harvard University Press, 1993.

Maxwell RJ. South Africa: A fragile miracle. *Lancet* 1995;345:1222–1224.

Mayer SE, Jencks C. Growing up in poor neighborhoods: How much does it matter? *Science* 1989;243:1441–1445.

McCalla S, Feldman J, Webbeh H et al. Changes in perinatal co- caine use in an inner city hospital, 1988 to 1992. *Am J Public Health* 1995;85:1695–1697.

McCord C, Freeman HP. Excess mortality in Harlem. *N Engl J Med* 1990;322:173–177.

McElvaine RS. *The Great Depression. America, 1929–1941*. New York, Random House, 1983, 1993.

McGinnis JM, Foege MH. Actual causes of death in the United States. *JAMA* 1993;270:2207–2212.

McGinnis JM, Lee PR. Healthy People 2000 at mid decade. *JAMA* 1995;273:1123–1129.

McKeown T. *The Modern Rise of Population*. London: Edward Arnold, 1976.

Michielutte R, Moore ML, Meis PJ, Ernest JM, Wells HB. Race differences in infant mortality from endogenous causes: A population-based study in North Carolina. *J Clin Epidemiol* 1994;47:119–130.

Miller CA. Wanting children. *Am J Public Health* 1992;82:341–343.

Mincy RB (ed). *Nurturing Young Black Males: Challenges to Agencies, Programs, and Social Policy*. Lanham, MD: The Urban Institute Press, 1993.

Montagu MFA. *Man's Most Dangerous Myth: The Fallacy of Race*. New York: Columbia University Press, 1941.

Morey RC, Ozcan YA, Retzlaff-Roberts DL et al. Estimating the hospital-wide cost differentials warranted for teaching hospitals. *Med Care* 1995;33:531–552.

Moy E, Bartman BA. Physician race and care of minority and medically indigent patients. *JAMA* 1995;273:1515–1520.

Murray C. *Losing Ground: American Social Policy, 1950–1980*. New York: Basic Books, 1984.

Myerberg DZ, Carpenter RG, Myerberg CF et al. Reducing postneonatal mortality in West Virginia: A statewide intervention program targeting risk identified at and after birth. *Am J Public Health* 1995;85:631–637.

Myrdal G. *An American Dilemma: The Negro Problem in Modern Democracy*. New York: Harper & Bros, 1944.

Myrdal G. *Challenge to Affluence*. New York: Pantheon, 1963.

Najman JM. Health and poverty: Past, present, and prospects for the future. *Soc Sci Med* 1993;36:157–166.

National Center for Health Statistics. *Vital Statistics of the United States, Vol. II, Section 6, Life Tables*. Washington, DC: U.S. Public Health Service, 1992.

National Center for Health Statistics. *Vital Statistics of the United States, 1987. Vol. III. Marriage and Divorce*. Hyattsville, MD: Public Health Service, 1991.

National Center for Health Statistics. *Health United States, 1992 and Healthy People 2000 Review*. Hyattsville, MD: Public Health Service, 1993.

National Center for Health Statistics. *Health United States, 1993*. Hyattsville, MD: Public Health Service, 1994.

Navarro V. Race or class versus race and class: Mortality differentials in the Unites States. *Lancet* 1990;2:1238–1240.

Nightingale EO. *Apartheid Medicine: Health and Human Rights in South Africa*. Washington, DC: American Association for the Advancement of Science, 1990.

Nightingale EO, Hannibal K, Geiger HJ et al. Apartheid medicine: Health and human rights in South Africa. *JAMA* 1990;264:2097–2102.

O'Campo P, Guyer B, Squires B et al. Needs assessment for reducing infant mortality in Baltimore City: The Healthy Start Program. *South Med J* 1993;86:1342–1349.

Orr ST, Charney E, Straus J. Use of health services by black children according to payment mechanism. *Med Care* 1988;26:939–947.

Osborne NG, Feit MD. The use of race in medical research. *JAMA* 1992;267:275–279.

Osterman P. Gains from growth? The impact of full employment on poverty in Boston.

In Jencks C, Peterson PE (eds): *The Urban Underclass.* Washington, DC: The Brookings Institution, 1991, pp 122–134.

Otten MW, Teutsch SM, Williamson DF, Marks JS. The effect of known risk factors on the excess mortality of black adults in the United States. *JAMA* 1990;263:845–850.

Ouellet RP, Apostolides AY, Entwistle G et al. Estimated community impact of hypertension control in a high risk population. *Am J Epidemiol* 1979;531–538.

Pappas G. Elucidating the relationships between race, socioeconomic status, and health. *Am J Public Health* 1994;84:892–893.

Pappas G. Queen A, Hadden Q et al. The increasing disparity in mortality between socioeconomic groups in the United States, 1960 and 1986. *N Engl J Med* 1993;329:103–109.

Parham D, Stephens D. Clinical preventive services in federally funded community and migrant health centers. In Proceedings of the 1991 Public Health Conference on Records and Statistics, Washington DC, 1992. Washington, DC: U.S. Government Printing Office, DHHS Publication No. PHS 92-1214, pp 361–364.

Parker RN. Poverty, subculture of violence, and type of homicide. *Social Forces* 1989;67:983–1007.

Parmer RJ, Stone RA, Cervenka JH. Renal hemodynamics in essential hypertension: Racial differences in response to changes in dietary sodium. *Hypertension* 1994;24:752–757.

Paschal A (ed). *W.E.B. Du Bois: A Reader.* New York: Macmillan, 1993, p 77.

Paul BK. Health service resources as determinants of infant death in rural Bangladesh: An empirical study. *Soc Sci Med* 1991;32:43–49.

Pauly MV, Danzon P, Feldstein PJ et al. *Responsible National Health Insurance.* Washington, DC: AEI Press, 1992.

Pearlin LI. The sociological study of stress. *J Health Soc Behav* 1989;30:241–256.

Peck MA. The importance of childhood socio-economic group for adult health. *Soc Sci Med* 1994:39:553–562.

Perez-Stabile EJ, Sabogal F, Otero-Sabrogal R et al. Misconceptions about cancer among Latinos and Anglos. *JAMA* 1992;268:3219–3223.

Peterson ED, Wright SM, Daly J, Thibault GE. Racial variation in cardiac procedure use and survival following acute myocardial infarction in the Department of Veterans Affairs. *JAMA* 1994;271:1175–1180.

Peterson GE (ed). *Big-City Politics, Governance, and Fiscal Constraints.* Washington, DC: Urban Institute Press, 1994.

Peterson PE. The urban underclass and the poverty paradox. In Jencks C, Peterson PE (eds): *The Urban Underclass.* Washington, DC: Brookings Institution, 1991, pp 3–27.

Perrucci R, Knudsen DD. *Sociology.* St. Paul, MN: West Publishing Co, 1983.

Pharoah POD, Morris JN. Postneonatal mortality. *Epidemiol Rev* 1979;1:170–183.

Plough A, Olafson F. Implementing the Boston Healthy Start initiative: A case study of community empowerment and public health. *Health Educ Q* 1994;21:221–234.

Polednak AP. *Racial and Ethnic Differences in Disease.* New York: Oxford University Press, 1989.

Polednak AP. Black–white differences in infant mortality in 38 Standard Metropolitan Statistical Areas. *Am J Public Health* 1991;81:1480–1482.

Polednak AP. Poverty, residential segregation, and black/white mortality rates in urban areas. *J Health Care Poor Underserv* 1993;4:363–373.

Polednak AP. Estimating smoking prevalence in Hispanic adults. *Health Values* 1994; 18:32–40.

Polednak AP. Trends in U.S. urban black infant mortality, by degree of segregation. *Am J Public Health* 1996a;86:723–726.

Polednak AP. Estimating mortality in the Hispanic population of Connecticut, 1990 to 1991. *Am J Public Health* 1995;85:998–1001.

Polednak AP. Segregation, discrimination and mortality in U.S. blacks. *Ethnicity Dis* 1996b;6:99–108.

Ponterotto JG, Pederson PB. *Preventing Prejudice: A Guide for Counselors and Educators.* Newbury Park, CA: Sage, 1993.

Priester R. A values framework for health system reform. *Health Affairs* 1992; Spring: 84–107.

Quadagno J. *The Color of Welfare.* New York: Oxford University Press, 1994.

Quillian L. Prejudice as a response to perceived group threat: Population composition and anti-immigrant and racial prejudice in Europe. *Am Sociol Rev* 1995;60:586–611.

Raczynski JM, Taykor H, Cutter G et al. Diagnoses, symptoms, and attribution of symptoms among black and white inpatients admitted for coronary heart disease. *Am J Public Health* 1994;84:951–956.

Rafferty MP. The effects of WIC and Medicaid participation on pregnancy outcome. Proceedings of the 1991 Public Health Conference on Records and Statistics. DHHS Publication No. PHS 92-1214. Washington, DC: U.S. Dept. of Health and Human Services, 1992.

Rank MR. *Living on the Edge: The Realities of Welfare in America.* New York: Columbia University Press, 1994.

Rawlings JS, Rawlings VB, Read JA. Prevention of low birth weight and preterm delivery in relation to interval between pregnancies among white and black women. *N Engl J Med* 1995;332:69–74.

Ray E. Struggle between young and old stunts NAACP growth (commentary). *Modern Maturity* 1995, Jan–Feb.

Reichman LB. How to ensure the continued resurgence of tuberculosis. *Lancet* 1996;347:175–177.

Richmond JA, Gaviria M, Flaherty JA et al. The process of acculturation: Theoretical perspectives and an empirical investigation in Peru. *Soc Sci Med* 1987;25:839–847.

Robins LN, Mills JL (eds). Effects of in utero exposure to street drugs. *Am J Public Health* 1993;83(Suppl):1–32.

Robinson JC. Exposure to occupational hazards among Hispanics, blacks, and non-Hispanic whites in California. *Am J Public Health* 1989;79:629–630.

Rogers RG. Living and dying in the U.S.A.: Sociodemographic determinants of death among blacks and whites. *Demography* 1992;29:287–303.

Romano PS, Bloom J, Syme SL. Smoking, social support, and hassles in an urban African-American community. *Am J Public Health* 1991;81:1415–1422.

Root MPP. *Racially Mixed People in the United States.* Newbury Park, CA: Sage, 1992.

Rosen SM. Achieving and sustaining full employment. *J Public Health Policy* 1995; 16:286–303.

Rosenbaum JE, Popkin SJ. Employment and earnings of low-income blacks who move to middle-class suburbs. In Jencks C, Peterson PE (eds): *The Urban Underclass.* Washington, DC: The Brookings Institution, 1992, pp 342–356.

Rowley D, Tosteson H. *Racial Differences in Preterm Delivery: Developing a New Paradigm*. New York: Oxford University Press, 1993.

Royce JM, Ashford A, Resnicow K et al. Physician- and nurse-assisted smoking cessation in Harlem. *J Natl Med Assoc* 1995;87:291–300.

Rutstein DD, Berenberg W, Chalmers TC et al. Measuring the quality of medical care. *N Engl J Med* 1976;294:582–588.

Sardell A. *The U.S. Experiment in Social Medicine: The Community Health Center Program, 1965–1986*. Pittsburgh: University of Pittsburgh Press, 1988.

Scherwitz LW, Perkins LL, Chesney MA et al. Hostility and health behaviors in young adults: The CARDIA study. *Am J Epidemiol* 1992;136:136–145.

Schneider D, Greenberg MR, Choi D. Black leaders' perceptions of the Year 2000 public health goals for black Americans. *Am J Public Health* 1993;83:1171–1173.

Schoendorf K, Hogue CJR, Kleinman JC, Rowley D. Mortality among infants of black as compared to white college-educated parents. *N Engl J Med* 1992;326:1522–1526.

Schuman H, Steeh C, Bobo L. *Racial Attitudes in America*. Cambridge, MA: Harvard University Press, 1985.

Schwartz E, Kofie VY, Rivo M, Tuckson RV. Black/white comparisons of deaths preventable by medical intervention: United States and the District of Columbia 1980–1986. *Int J Epidemiol* 1990;19:591–598.

Schwarz JE, Volgy TJ. *The Forgotten Americans*. New York: Norton, 1992.

Scribner R, Hohn A, Dwyer J. Blood pressure and self-concept among African-Americans. *J Natl Med Assoc* 1995;87:417–422.

Shea S, Misra D, Erhlich MH et al. Correlates of nonadherence to hypertension treatment in an inner-city minority population. *Am J Public Health* 1992a;82:1607–1612.

Shea S, Misra D, Erhlich MH et al. Predisposing factors for severe, uncontrolled hypertension in an inner-city minority population. *N Engl J Med* 1992b;327:776–781.

Sherwood A, May CW, Siegel WC et al. Ethnic differences in hemodynamic responses to stress in hypertensive men and women. *Am J Hypertens* 1995;8:552–557.

Shiono PH, Klebanoff MA, Graubard BI et al. Birth weight among women of different ethnic groups. *JAMA* 1986;255:48–52.

Siegler IC, Peterson BL, Barefoot JC. Hostility during late adolescence predicts coronary risk factors at mid-life. *Am J Epidemiol* 1992;136:146–154.

Silver GA. Virchow, the heroic model in medicine: Health policy by accolade. *Am J Public Health* 1987;77:82–88.

Singh GK, Yu SM. Infant mortality in the United States: Trends, differentials and projections, 1950 through 2010. *Am J Public Health* 1995;85:957–964.

Smith GD, Egger M. Socioeconomic differences in mortality in Britain and the United States. *Am J Public Health* 1992;82:1168–1170.

Somova LI, Connolly C, Diara K. Psychosocial predictors of hypertension in black and white Africans. *J Hypertens* 1995;13:193–199.

Sorlie PD, Backlund E, Johnson NJ et al. Mortality by Hispanic status in the United States. *JAMA* 1993;270:2464–2468.

Sorlie PD, Backlund E, Keller JB. U.S. mortality by economic, demographic and social characteristics: The National Longitudinal Mortality Study. *Am J Public Health* 1995;85:949–956.

Sorlie P, Rogot E, Anderson R, Johnson NJ, Backlund E. Black–white mortality differences by family income. *Lancet* 1992;340:346–350.

St. John C, Bates NA. Racial composition and neighborhood evaluation. *Soc Sci Res* 1989;19:47–61.

Stafford WW, Ladner J. Political dimensions of the underclass concept. In Gans HJ (ed): *Sociology in America.* Newbury Park, CA: Sage Publications, 1990, pp. 138–155.

Stearns LB, Logan JR. The racial structuring of the housing market and segregation in suburban areas. *Soc Forces* 1986;65:28–42.

Steinberg S. *The Ethnic Myth: Race, Ethnicity, and Class in America.* Boston, MA: Beacon, 1989, p 293.

Stevens G, Swicegood G. The linguistic context of ethnic endogamy. *Am Sociol Rev* 1987;52:73–82.

Stout NA, Jenkins L, Pizatella TJ. Occupational injury mortality rates in the United States: Changes from 1980 to 1989. *Am J Public Health* 1996;86:73–77.

Struening EL, Wallace R, Moore R. Housing conditions and the quality of children at birth. *Bull NY Acad Med* 1990;66:463–478.

Stuckey S. *Slave Culture.* New York: Oxford University Press, 1987.

Sullivan EA, Kreiswirth BN, Palumbo L et al. Emergence of fluoroquinolone-resistance tuberculosis in New York City. *Lancet* 1995;345:1148–1150.

Sundquist J. Ethnicity, social class and health. A population-based study of the influence of social factors on self-reported illness in 223 Latin American refugees, 333 Finnish and 126 South European labour migrants and 841 Swedish controls. *Soc Sci Med* 1995;40:777–787.

Sung JFC, Coates RJ, Williams JE et al. Cancer screening intervention among blacks women in inner-city Atlanta—Design of a study. *Public Health Rep* 1992; 107381–388.

Susser E, Moore R, Link B. Risk factors for homelessness. *Epidemiol Rev* 1993;15:547–556.

Susser M. Apartheid and the causes of death: Disentangling ideology and laws from class and race. *Am J Public Health* 1983;73:581–584.

Susser M. *Sociology in Medicine.* New York: Oxford University Press,1985.

Sutton GF. Assessing mortality and morbidity disadvantages of the black population of the United States. *Soc Biol* 1971;369–383.

Targonski PV, Persky VW, Orris P et al. Trends in asthma mortality among African Americans and whites in Chicago, 1968 through 1991. *Am J Public Health* 1994;84:1830–1833.

Telles EE. Residential segregation by skin color in Brazil. *Am Sociol Rev* 1992;57:186–197.

Thomas SB, Quinn SC. The Tuskegee syphilis study, 1932 to 1972: Implications for HIV education and AIDS risk education programs in the black community. *Am J Public Health* 1991;81:1498–1504.

Thomas SM, Quinn SC, Billingsley A et al. The characteristics of northern black churches with community health outreach programs. *Am J Public Health* 1994;84:575–579.

Tienda M, Stier H. Joblessness and shiftlessness: Labor force activity in Chicago's inner city. In Jencks C, Peterson PE (eds): *The Urban Underclass.* 1991, Washington, DC: Brookings Institution, pp 135–154.

Tilson HH Jr, Ross M, Calkins D. Medicaid and Medicare. In Calkins D, Fernandopulle RJ, Marino BS (eds): *Health Care Policy.* Cambridge, MA: Blackwell Science, 1995, pp 102–121.

Townsend P. Widening inequalities of health in Britain: A rejoinder to Rudolph Klein. *Int J Health Services* 1990;20:363–372.

Tucker MB, Mitchell-Kernan C (eds): *The Decline in Marriage among African Americans*. New York: Russell Sage Foundation, 1995.

Turner LW, Sutherland M, Harris GJ et al. Cardiovascular health promotion in North Florida African-American churches. *Health Values* 1995;19:3–9.

U.S. Bureau of the Census. *Poverty in the United States: 1990*. Current Population Reports, Consumer Income Series P-60, No. 175, 1991a.

U.S. Bureau of the Census. *Trends in Relative Income: 1964 to 1989*. Current Population Reports, Consumer Income, Series P-60, No. 177, 1991b.

U.S. Bureau of the Census. Current Population Reports, P70-31. *Characteristics of Recipients and the Dynamics of Program Participation: 1987–1988 (Selected Data from the Survey of Income and Program Participation)*. Washington, DC: U.S. Government Printing Office, 1992a.

U.S. Bureau of the Census. *Statistical Abstract of the United States: 1992*. 112th Ed. Washington, DC, U.S. Government Printing Office, 1992b.

U.S. Bureau of the Census. *Money Income of Households, Families, and Persons in the United States: 1992*. Current Population Reports, Series P60-184. Washington, DC: U.S. Government Printing Office, 1993.

U.S. Bureau of the Census. *Statistical Abstract of the United States: 1994*. Washington, DC: U.S. Government Printing Office, 1994.

U.S. Bureau of the Census. Census Bureau releases information on income, poverty, and health insurance coverage in 1994. *U.S. Department of Commerce News*. Press release, October 5, 1995.

U.S. Deptartment of Health and Human Services. *Healthy People 2000: National Health and Disease Objectives*. DHHS Publication No. (PHS) 91-50212. Washington, DC: U.S. Department of Health and Human Services, 1991.

Vagero D. Inequality in health—Some theoretical and empirical problems. *Soc Sci Med* 1991;32:367–371.

Valdez RB, Morgenstern H, Brown ER et al: Insuring Latinos against the costs of illness. *JAMA* 1993;269:889–894.

Vergara CJ. *The New American Ghetto*. New Brunswick, NJ: Rutgers University Press, 1995.

Vernon SW, Buffler PA. The status of status inconsistency. *Epidemiol Rev* 1988;10:65–85.

Vital Statistics of the United States. Mortality, Part B. Hyattsville, MD: U.S. Department of Health and Human Services. Multiple volumes, 1982–1990a.

Vital Statistics of the United States. Natality. Hyattsville, MD: U.S. Department of Health and Human Services. Multiple volumes, 1982–1990b.

Wagner-Echeagaray FA, Schutz CG, Chilcoat HD et al. Degree of acculturation and the risk of crack cocaine smoking among Hispanic American. *Am J Public Health* 1994;84:1825–1827.

Walcott-McQuigg JA. The relationship between stress and weight-control behavior in African-American women. *J Natl Med Assoc* 1995;87:427–432.

Wallace D. Roots of increased health care inequality in New York. *Soc Sci Med* 1990;31:1219–1227.

Wallace D. The resurgence of tuberculosis in New York City: A mixed hierarchically and spatially diffused epidemic. *Am J Public Health* 1994;84:1000–1002.

Wallace R, Wallace D. Origins of public health collapse in New York City: The dynamics of planned shrinkage, contagious urban decay and social disintegration. *Bull NY Acad Med* 1990;66:391–434.

Washburn RA, Kline G, Lackland DT et al. Leisure time physical activity: Are there black/white differences? *Prev Med* 1992;21:127–135.

Washington JM (ed). *I Have a Dream: Writings and Speeches that Changed the World. Martin Luther King, Jr.* New York: HarperCollins, 1992, p 187.

Watson SD. Minority access and health reform: A civil right to health care. *J Law Medicine Ethics* 1994;22:127–137.

Weatherall D. *The Role of Medical Research in Health Care.* New York: WW Norton, 1995.

Weicher JC. A new war on poverty: The Kemp program to empower the poor. In Darby MR (ed): *Reducing Poverty in America.* Thousand Oaks, CA: Sage, 1996, pp 199–223.

Weinrich SP, Weinrich MC, Keil JE, Gazes PC, Potter E. The John Henryism and Framingham type A scales. *Am J Epidemiol* 1988;128:165–178.

Weitzman BC, Knikman JR, Shinn M. Predictors of shelter use among low-income families: Psychiatric history, substance abuse, and victimization. *Am J Public Health* 1992;82:1547–1550.

West C. *Race Matters.* New York: Vintage, 1994.

Wildey MB, Young RL, Elder JP et al. Cigarette point-of-sale advertising in ethnic neighborhoods in San Diego, California. *Heath Values* 1992;16:23–28.

Wilkinson RG. National mortality rates: The impact of inequality? *Am J Public Health* 1992;82:1082–1084.

Williams DR, Lavizzo-Mourey R, Warren RC. The concept of race and health status is America. *Public Health Rep* 1994;109:26–41.

Williams DR, Lepkowski JM. Poverty and health: A national study of the determinants of excess mortality. PHS Publication No. 92-1214.Washington, DC: U.S. Government Printing Office, 1992, pp 217–222.

Williams RR, Hunt SC, Hasstedt SJ et al. Are there interactions and relations between genetic and environmental factors predisposing to high blood pressure? *Hypertension* 1991;18(Suppl. I):I29–I37.

Williams T, Kornblum W. Public housing projects as successful environments for adolescent development. *Ann NY Acad Sci* 1995;749:153–177.

Wilson TW, Hollifoeld LR, Grim CE. Systolic blood pressure levels in black populations in sub-Sahara Africa, the West Indies, and the United States: A meta-analysis. *Hypertension* 1991;18(Suppl. I):I87–I91.

Wilson WJ. *The Truly Disadvantaged.* Chicago: University of Chicago Press, 1987.

Wilson WJ. Public policy research and "The Truly Disadvantaged." In Jencks C, Peterson PE (eds): *The Urban Underclass.* Washington, DC: Brooking Institution, 1991a, pp 460–481.

Wilson WJ. Studying inner-city dislocations: The challenge of public agenda research. *Am Sociol Rev* 1991b;56:1–14.

Winkleby MA, Fortmann SP, Barrett DC. Social class disparities in risk factors for disease: Eight-year prevalence patterns by level of education. *Prev Med* 1990;19:1–12.

Winkleby MA, Jatulis DE, Frank E et al. Socioeconomic status and health: How education, income, and occupation contribute to risk factors for disease. *Am J Public Health* 1992a;82:816–820.

Winkleby MA, Rockhill B, Jatulis D et al. The medical origins of homelessness. *Am J Public Health* 1992b;83:1395–1398.

Wise PH, Pursley DM. Infant mortality as a social mirror. *N Engl J Med* 1992;326:1558–1560.

Woodruff SI, Agro AD, Wildey MB et al. Point-of-purchase tobacco advertising: Prevalence, correlates, and a brief intervention. *Health Values* 1995;19:56–62.

Woolhandler S, Himmelstein DU, Silber R, Bader M, Harnly M, Jones AA. Medical care and mortality: Racial differences in preventable deaths. *Int J Health Serv* 1989;15:1–11.

World Health Organization (WHO). *Apartheid and Health.* Geneva: WHO, 1983.

Yankauer A. The relationship of fetal and infant mortality to residential segregation. *Am Sociol Rev* 1950;15:644–648.

Yankauer A. The deadliest plague. *Am J Public Health* 1989;79:821–822.

Yankauer A. What infant mortality tells us. *Am J Public Health* 1990;80:653–654.

Zigler E, Piotrkoswki CS, Collins R. Health services in Head Start. *Annu Rev Public Health* 1994;15:311–334.

Zigler E, Styfco SJ. Reshaping early childhood interventions to be a more effective weapon against poverty. In Darby MR (ed): *Reducing Poverty in America.* Thousand Oaks, CA: Sage, 1996, pp 310–333.

Index